D0341455

PRAISE FOR *BACKBONE*

"My friend Karen Duffy, who lives with unimaginable pain, has taught me so much; that my complaints are the most ridiculous in the world."

—George Clooney

"Writing from the heart and the funny bone, Duff shares her raw and inspiring triumph over extreme pain and illness. Her bone-deep understanding of how to transcend suffering is a must-read. Thank you, Duff, for shedding light on the pathway to empowered living."

—Dr. Beth Darnall, author of *Less Pain, Fewer Pills: Avoid the Dangers of Prescription Opioids and Gain Control Over Chronic Pain* and *The Opioid-Free Pain Relief Kit*

"It's highly beneficial to have a book that brings hope and humor to people. *Backbone* is inspiring and alive, a rare book that offers insight for the patient and the people who love them."

—Ginger Spitzer, Executive Director, Foundation for Sarcoidosis Research

"Karen Duffy may just be the world's finest alchemist. Her bodacious, brilliant, joyous—yes JOYOUS—book about chronic pain isn't just one of the best memoirs I've ever read, it's one of the best books I've ever read in my lifetime. Full of witty wisdoms, it's an unputdownable triumph of the spirit. I just love this book!"

—Marisa Acocella Marchetto, author of *Cancer Vixen*

"*Backbone* is beautifully written, laugh out funny, and profoundly moving. It will charm and delight, the interactive graphics are brilliant. I'm wearing the 'I Got Out of Bed Today Crown' as I write this review. I cannot recommend this book more highly."

—Carole Radziwill, Emmy Award–winning producer and author of the *New York Times* bestseller *What Remains*

"*Backbone* is an owner's manual for anyone whose body is behaving badly. Sensible, inspirational, and above all, hilarious. It's like sharing a hospital room with Nora Ephron."

—Edward Conlon, bestselling author of *Blue Blood*

"*Backbone* is amazing. It is a memoir of sorts—chronic pain meets hysterical laughter. Even though it's a book of how Duff lives with pain, each page is a surprise. With *Backbone*, she's written a book for people who are sick and people who share a sick sense of humor."

—Tabitha Soren, photographer and author of *Fantasy Life*

"*Backbone* . . . gives a new and strangely inspiring spin to Samuel Beckett's maxim, 'Nothing is funnier than unhappiness.' With grace and great humor, Duffy records her endurance of considerable and prolonged suffering only to reveal, through her example, how that can be diminished and marginalized in a life invested with gratitude and determination. This book should be given to all chronic complainers to cure them of their ailment."

—Christopher Cahill, Director of the American Irish Historical Society

BACKBONE

KAREN DUFFY

BACKBONE

LIVING WITH CHRONIC PAIN
WITHOUT TURNING INTO ONE

Arcade Publishing • New York

First Edition

Arcade Publishing books may be purchased in bulk at special discounts for sales promotion, corporate gifts, fund-raising, or educational purposes. Special editions can also be created to specifications. For details, contact the Special Sales Department, Arcade Publishing, 307 West 36th Street, 11th Floor, New York, NY 10018 or arcade@skyhorsepublishing.com.

Arcade Publishing® is a registered trademark of Skyhorse Publishing, Inc.®, a Delaware corporation.

Visit our website at www.arcadepub.com.

10 9 8 7 6 5 4 3 2 1

Duffy, Karen, author.
Backbone : living with chronic pain without turning into one / Karen Duffy.
First edition. | New York : Arcade Publishing, [2017]
Identifiers: LCCN 2017032495 (print) | LCCN 2017036047 (ebook) | ISBN 9781628727968 (Ebook) | ISBN 9781628727951 (hardcover : alk. paper)
Subjects: LCSH: Duffy, Karen, ---Health. | Sarcoidosis--Patients--Biography. | Chronic pain--Patients--Biography. | Chronic pain--Humor.
Classification: LCC RC182.S14 (ebook) | LCC RC182.S14 D83 2017 (print) | DDC 616.4/290092 [B] --dc23

Cover design by Brian Peterson

Image on page xii courtesy of Wong-Baker FACES Foundation (2017). Wong-Baker FACES® Pain Rating Scale. Retrieved 7/26/2017 with permission from http://www.Wong-BakerFACES.org.

Image on page 230 is reprinted from the *Journal of Psychosomatic Research*, 11/2, Holmes, Thomas H., and Richard H. Rahe, The social readjustment rating scale. 213-18, Copyright 1967, with permission from Elsevier.

Printed in the United States of America

For John Fortune Lambros and Jack Augustine Lambros.

"There is not a particle of my love that is not yours."
—James Joyce

I believe that much of a man's character will be found betokened in his backbone.

—Herman Melville, *Moby Dick*

CONTENTS

INTRODUCTION

I HAVE A CHRONIC illness called sarcoidosis of the central nervous system. It's a multi-system inflammatory disease of unknown origin. A healthy immune system defends your body from disease; with sarcoidosis, the immune system is what's causing the problem. My body is making itself sick. Sarcoidosis causes the immune system to create inflammatory lesions called granulomas. I have cultivated a bumper crop of these granulomas in my brain, central nervous system, and lungs. They can attack any organ. Only my teeth and hair are not targets for more lesions.

When I first got sick, I thought the doctors would figure it out and I'd get better and go back to my life the way it was before. It didn't turn out that way. The disease has irreparably damaged my central nervous system. I never imagined that the pain was going to last this long, that it would be endless, and that I'd have to figure out how to deal with it for the rest of my life.

Over 115 million Americans live with chronic pain. "Chronic" means it lasts anywhere from twelve weeks to life. When one third of all Americans are dealing with long-term pain, you'd think there would be some kind of massive medical effort to deal with it, like with cancer, smoking, and obesity. But instead, you've got this book.

Storytelling is a natural reaction to illness, or so it seems if you look at all the memoirs written by people who got sick. We write to make sense of life, and illness interrupts the story of our lives. The trouble with "sickness books" is they often try too hard to inspire you. Sometimes they can read as more inspirational than believable. A catastrophic illness can't always be equated to a great spiritual awakening.

This isn't a misery memoir or a self-help book. But I hope it does help you. I recognize that what works for me isn't necessarily going to work for you. I won't bully you with positivity. I give you, the reader, too much credit and respect to boss you around when you're kind enough to crack open my book.

I wrote a book about getting through the acute stage of my illness, titled *Model Patient: My Life as an Incurable Wise-Ass.* I have now lived with the consequences of chronic sarcoidosis for many years, and I realized there was more to say.

I've learned a lot from my illness. In some ways, it has been a gift. It's not a gift I would have picked out for myself, but when things were easy, I didn't realize how tough I was. When you live with chronic illness, you get comfortable with being uncomfortable. There is an upside to having your life turned upside down.

If I were to give you just one piece of advice, it's this: pain is inevitable, but suffering is optional. Be the best person you can be, because that is what transforms a sufferer into an endurer.

If I were to give you *two* pieces of advice, the second one would be to finish this book. I've done my best to make it entertaining and useful, whether you're sick or just have a sick sense of humor.

- -

THE BILL MURRAY-KAREN DUFFY
PAIN RATING SCALE

The Wong-Baker FACES Pain Rating scale is a visual aid to help a patient rate her pain level. It was created for children, but is now used around the world for anyone over the age of three.

While I like the idea, I think there might be a more relatable way to calibrate a pain scale. Mark Twain remarked that the only way to cheer yourself up is to cheer someone else up; Bill Murray (who recently won the Mark Twain Prize for American Humor) is a friend who cheers me immensely. I think seeing his handsome kisser on a pain scale instead of infantile smiley faces will cheer you up too.

- -

Wong-Baker FACES® Pain Rating Scale

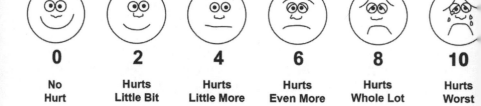

0	2	4	6	8	10
No Hurt	Hurts Little Bit	Hurts Little More	Hurts Even More	Hurts Whole Lot	Hurts Worst

Instructions for Usage

Explain to the person that each face represents a person who has no pain (hurt), or some, or a lot of pain.

Face 0 doesn't hurt at all. Face 2 hurts just a little bit. Face 4 hurts a little bit more. Face 6 hurts even more. Face 8 hurt a whole lot. Face 10 hurts as much as you can imagine, although you don't have to be crying to have this worst pain.

Ask the person to choose the face that best depicts the pain they are experiencing.

Originally published in *Whaley & Wong's Nursing Care of Infants and Children.*

© Elsevier Inc.

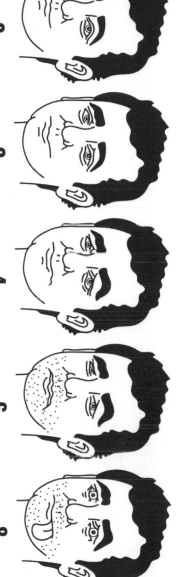

THE DUFFY/MURRAY PAIN SCALE

0 — YOU'RE AWESOME

2 — YOU'RE AWESOME
but this smarts!

4 — YOU'RE AWESOME
but cheese on a cracker
this hurts!

6 — YOU'RE AWESOME
but this excruciating sensation is
vexing me sorely!

8 — YOU'RE AWESOME
but this disagreeable feeling is
causing me quite a bit of distress.

10 — YOU'RE AWESOME
I'm awesome, but this the worst
pain imaginable! I'm not joking!

THE ECCEDENTESIAST

THERE IS PAIN THAT hurts you and pain that changes you. Acute physical pain is a signal and a survival mechanism. In the short term it compels you to do something to avoid or diminish it—pull your hand away from the hot stove, jump back from a prickly cactus. Acute pain is usually caused by tissue damage and will resolve over a period of less than three months. It hurts, but it will go away. You'll get better. You'll go back to being the person you were before.

When your condition progresses from acute to chronic and the pain becomes permanent, this is the pain that changes you. There is physical pain, but there may be no visible injury. It's inside, in the nervous system. It is invisible. The nerves never stop firing, sending constant pain signals to your brain. You can't jump back from this pain. It follows you, and you have no choice but to reach an accommodation with it. You can medically dull it or mentally distract yourself from it, but you can never escape chronic pain.

The International Association for the Study of Pain has proposed this definition for pain: "an unpleasant sensory and emotional experience, associated with actual or potential tissue damage." There is a major emotional component to dealing with chronic pain, but right now I'm just talking about the physical aspect. The pain I endure is called neuropathic pain, which means it's caused by damage to the nerves themselves, not to the surrounding tissue. According to the editor of PAIN, the *Journal of the International Association for the Study of Pain*, neuropathic pain is the most excruciating pain of all. I could have told him that myself and saved him the money he spent on his PhD.

The English word "pain" is rooted in the Latin "poena," meaning "punishment" and "penalty," as well as the sensation one feels when hurt. Chronic pain is like serving a life sentence. It's punishment for a crime you didn't commit.

One of the punitive effects of pain is that it is unshareable—it is difficult or impossible to express. To the sufferer, the pain cannot be denied. To the person next to her, the pain cannot be confirmed. Pain is subjective. It is unknowable unless you are afflicted with it. We tend to deny the pain of others because we can't see it or feel it. It's mystifying to us, unreal and frightening. We don't want it to be true because we all fear being in pain. Pain means illness. Illness means limits and loss of freedom. If we admit someone else's suffering, we admit the possibility that we might suffer too. And yet one-third of Americans has some type of chronic pain. That's over 115 million people (all of whom I expect to buy this book), more than the number of people who suffer from heart disease and diabetes combined. So why is it so hard for us to talk about pain?

In *The Body in Pain*, Harvard professor Elaine Scarry writes that "physical pain does not simply resist language, but actively destroys it." She studied the effects of severe and prolonged pain and noted that "pain is resistant to lingual expression," and this is part of the isolation that pain sufferers endure. A person in pain is bereft of the resource of language. She cites Virginia Woolf, who wrote, "English, which can express the thoughts of Hamlet and the tragedy of Lear has no words for the shiver and the headache . . . the merest schoolgirl, when she falls in love, has Shakespeare or Keats to speak her mind for her; but let a sufferer try to describe a pain in his head to a doctor and language at once runs dry."

Pain can reduce language, and the difficulty in describing it can compound the loneliness of a chronic condition. Because pain is so difficult to express, doctors at McGill University in Canada have created a questionnaire to help describe the severity of pain (you will find information and a link to the questionnaire on page 231). It is seventy-eight questions long, and on the basis of your answers, it gives you seven words to describe the pain to your doctor. This is useful when you need medical help. But it's not so helpful when answering the everyday question from a friend, "How are you feeling?"

Physical pain is isolating. Its inexpressibility and incomprehensibility separates you from your family and friends. My husband and son have no idea what it is like to live with chronic pain. They're loving, funny, and compassionate, and they are essentially healthy. They, like most people, have a narrow frame of reference for how to comprehend pain. Their sprains and stitches and dental visits are finite, a sprint through pain. My chronic pain is an unending marathon of physical distress. They can't see the agony of the evil parrot perched on my shoulder, digging his sharp scaly claws into my shoulder and pecking my head and neck with its razor-blade beak. The torment that bursts in my neck and ruptures through my central nervous system is invisible.

From the moment I wake, before I even open my eyes, the pain detonates on the right side of my head, from the top of my ear through to my neck and shoulder. Then it jumps down my spinal column and over to my left elbow, igniting a searing, burning sensation that makes my left hand contract into a sad claw, a collapsed fist of fingers. Then the intense nerve jangling vibrates down my spinal column to my feet, where both my big toes feel like they have been snapped into a pair of rat traps. I'm amazed that my guys cannot see the raw pain in my body. How is it not visible? How can it not radiate out of me like the little jagged lines and stars emanating from an injured cartoon character?

The toughest part of my day is waking in the morning, arising with pain, swallowing, and then waiting for the medicine to kick in. It's like waking up with a hangover, but I didn't have the fun of getting hammered the night before.

When the pain is at its worst, my head is tilted to the right like a broken Pez dispenser. I cannot tolerate the lightest touch; even wind will sting my neck. When air hurts, it is termed allodynia, meaning a painful reaction caused by a stimulus that would not normally cause pain. Sensations from showering, wearing a collared shirt, having hair strands brush against my neck, or even a light breeze can cause allodynia. Most pain serves a purpose, to protect an injured area. Allodynia flares pain for no useful purpose.

I take prescription medications to tamp down the burning, biting sharp sensations. Before the medicine takes effect, it feels like a donkey wearing hockey skates is kicking me in the neck. After the medication, it feels like the jackass put skate guards on, but he's still kicking.

My vocabulary at these times consists of "ouch," "yeow," and "UGH!" Using profanity actually has a demonstrated palliative effect, but I'm not much of a curser.

Not long ago, I was heading out to the patio to put sausages on the grill. The neuropathy in my feet impairs my spatial awareness, and I stubbed my foot on an Adirondack chair so hard that I broke two bones in my left foot. (I also dropped all the sausages.) My husband drove me to the hospital, and when the doctor reset the bone back into place, it was one of the most painful things I'd ever experienced. I couldn't help screaming, but I didn't want to swear because there was a little kid in the ER. The doctor told me afterwards I was yelling "Mahatma Gandhi! Mahatma Gandhi!"

Other than talking about my pain, there's really no way for people to know I'm seriously ill. You'll see my defensive stance, ready to avoid anything that might touch the hot zone. You will not see my affliction. The granulomas and lesions are knotted up my spinal cord and in my central nervous system. I have an invisible illness.

I know that a lot of you reading this are living with chronic pain, too. My hope is that this book will help relieve the isolation and perhaps help you feel understood and connected. Chronic pain is the number one cause of disability in the United States, so you're not alone. Nearly one third of Americans live with chronic pain.

An eccedentesiast is someone who hides her misery behind a big fat smile, and that's my approach to pain. I think it's better than grimacing in agony, and there's evidence that the act of smiling actually makes you happier. It's frustrating that I can't share my pain, but I'm trying to share my joy instead. As

Lord Byron advised, "Always laugh when you can, it's cheap medicine."

Living with a degenerative disease is like living next door to a bully. You never know when he's going to come over and ring your bell and knock you on your keister. Sarcoidosis is a part of me, and I am doing my best to peacefully cohabitate with it. I try to keep the pain-to-fun ratio leaning in my favor, and this is how I go on—smiling through the pain, trying to find a bright side. Every day I have a choice: to be useful or useless. I choose to be useful, or I try to, and this contributes to my happiness. I've had more than my share in the past fifteen years. In a way, I think I am a very lucky unlucky person.

THE ECCEDENTESIAST MASK

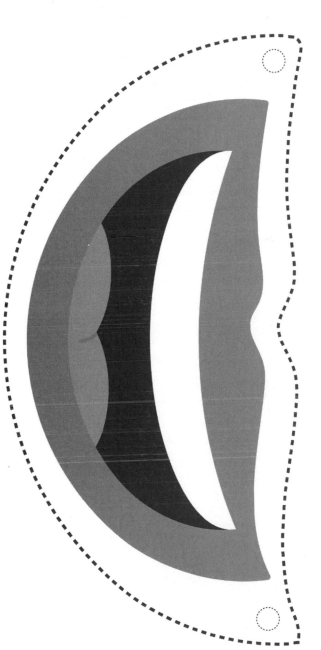

HOW TO MAKE YOUR ECCEDENTESIAST MASK.

1. Cut along the dotted line.
2. Punch hole on either side and thread through ribbon.

GETTING OLD FOR THE THIRD TIME

I DON'T FEEL BAD about my neck. I feel pain, because my neck hurts, badly. I *do* feel bad that looking your age can be considered a negative. It's crazy to view getting old as undesirable. It is a luxury that is not guaranteed to everyone.

It's said that life begins at forty, but that's also when it begins to show. Bette Davis famously said that "getting old isn't for sissies." She was right on, and I should know, because this is the third time I'm getting old.

I thought aging was a slow process. Gradually the years and experience pile on, and with imperceptible slowness, time begins to tell and your face fills up with "character." Age doesn't creep up on you; it hits you like a bus. Your physical prime is finite. Time may bring wisdom, but it's one hell of a lousy beautician. All at once it's goodbye to the tomboyish gamine you used to see in the mirror, and hello Ernest Borgnine! Inside every middle-aged woman is her younger self, wondering, "What the hell just happened?"

The first time I got old was in my mid-twenties. I was employed as a recreational therapist at a nursing home. My job was to perk up the old folks: organize art classes, call bingo games, and host the Frank Sinatra Appreciation Club. I loved my job, and the confidence I felt from being a successful rec-reational therapist gave me the bravery to take the leap and send in an unsolicited audition tape to MTV.

To everyone's surprise, including mine, I landed a coveted job as an MTV VJ (video jockey). I had experience with an audience that had a two-inch attention span. My skill set with distracted spectators worked in my favor. MTV was blamed for shortening the attention span of our adolescent audience, but I preferred to think that they were becoming more like their elders.

It was the dawn of the grunge era, and the viewers of the channel were mainly zit-spangled teenage boys rebelling in flannel and musty thrift-shop sweaters. My esteemed col-leagues were just out of college; I was a grown woman who'd had a successful career as a healthcare professional. And now I'd gone from documenting protocols for the care of the elderly to dressing in miniskirts and conducting interviews backstage at U2 concerts. Around the old folks I felt young; around the MTV audience I felt, suddenly, old. I felt like mutton dressed as lamb.

I did not take a traditional career trajectory, but some peo-ple are born to push the envelope and some were born to lick it. I taught myself some memorization techniques so I didn't have to rely on a TelePrompTer or cue cards. I took prepara-tion seriously and worked hard to make it look easy. I had a blast, and many of my closest friendships began at MTV when I was the new girl.

I'd found my métier. I enjoyed the challenge of writing and hosting TV programs. I was a bit long in the tooth to be an ingénue, but I lucked out, and Revlon Cosmetics signed me to a multi-year contract as a spokesmodel.

I was also beginning to get cast in major films, but here I rose to my level of incompetence. As an actress, my emotive range was fabulously narrow. I was wooden and overwhelmed. Looking back, my presence was so weak it's a miracle that it even stuck to the film. I would not watch one of my old films if it were screening on my own corneas. If you poisoned me and hid the antidote in a copy of the Disney movie I was in called *Blank Check*, I'd say my goodbyes now. I should have been arrested for criminally bad acting. But despite the poor quality of my on-screen performance, it was an exciting, thrilling, and crazy-busy time of my life.

The second time I got old wasn't nearly as much fun. In my early thirties I was diagnosed with a rare disease, sarcoidosis of the central nervous system. Getting sick isn't for sissies, either.

All of a sudden, I was too debilitated to continue working. It was like I had been building an airplane by hand, and when I was finally ready to take off, I had to lock it up in a hangar. Good-bye to the camaraderie of living on location and being interviewed on late-night TV, hello to bedsores and becoming barren. I went through a very early mid-life crisis at thirty-three. I had to mourn for my old life and figure out how to live this new one. At least sarcoidosis spared the world from any more Karen Duffy films—I had signed a three-picture deal with a major studio right before I got sick. I shudder to think what might have been.

Sarcoidosis is a complicated inflammatory disorder. My body was attacking itself from the inside out. There is no cure, and the side effects of the treatment can be deadly. The chemotherapy drug I took for six years kills fast-growing cells. Another drug I was taking launched me into a medical menopause. I was in the prime of my baby-making years and had to put fertility on hold. The fun was never-ending.

One drug made me lose the hair on my head and another gave me a mustache. I was the only Revlon model who could have filmed a convincing advertising campaign for after-shave. You know how Eskimos have one hundred words for snow? I found an old Albanian-English dictionary, and the Albanians have twenty-seven words for eyebrows and twenty-seven words for mustache. In Albanian, *mustaqe pasht* means a droopy Wilfred Brimley style 'stache. It seems like facial hair plays an important role in Albanian culture. Too bad I'm not Albanian.

In Farsi, the word "mahji" means looking beautiful after a disease, which I found encouraging. My illness became my metamorphosis. It took seven years of chemo drugs and long hospital visits to get my disease to a manageable and chronic condition. I learned to exist with sarcoidosis and created a whole new life. I'm still sick, but my doctor says I look a lot better in person than I do on paper.

Day to day, chronic pain is my biggest issue. The only medic alert bracelet I have is a joke one from my friend Francis. He had it engraved to announce that my condition is that I'm a "Sick F***."

The years of acute illness weren't all bad. I eloped with my husband when I was still in the catastrophically ill stage. John had heard I was quite sick, and he bought me a dog bed so I had a comfortable place to lie on the bathroom floor when I was suffering the nauseating side effects of my drug protocol. We had met years earlier, and I was always crazy about him. There is nothing like the pointy edge of mortality to encourage you to take a leap to matrimony. Getting married was a big part of getting old for the second time, a good part.

Hypergamy is where you marry up, and I hit the jackpot with John. He's smart and funny and handsome and is the best partner I could ever imagine. It's a mixed marriage. I'm from a scrappy middle-class Irish Catholic family, and he is a prep school, Ivy League financial investor from the Upper East Side. I'm sick, and he's intensely healthy. We share different histories but similar values. We promised to always treat each other with respect, and we make a great team. He's the only person who can consistently crack me up. Aristotle thought that spouses hold up a mirror to each other. I guess both John and I like what we see. In the Olympics of love, I got the gold medal. In a zombie apocalypse, we could anticipate each other's actions. I bet together we could kill an army of zombies, if zombies actually died.

Now I'm getting old for the third time, and this time, it's for real. To my surprise, it's a lot more fun than it looks. Age is the sum of all the choices we have made, how we've lived our lives and how we think about the future. You can't change your chronological age, but how you age is up to you.

WHEN ARE YOU OLD?

Dante Alighieri, the author of the *Inferno*, said that old age begins at forty-five, which seems on the early side. According to the American Association of Retired Persons, it's fifty—that's when they send you the membership card, which is nice for the discounts, but a lot of people just start hitting their stride at fifty (I hope I did). The United Nations says old age begins at sixty, but they're taking into account all the people around the world who have struggled with manual labor their whole lives just to make a dollar a day. By the time these hardworking souls make sixty, they are old. I hope that these people are able to enjoy a better standard of living, one that leaves them wondering when, exactly, after five decades of life, old age starts. I don't have any definitive answer, but I intend to spend many years finding out.

- -

Our culture is terrified of becoming old. The composer Igor Stravinsky described aging—erroneously, I believe—as "the ever shrinking perimeter of pleasure." I think this attitude persists partly because older people don't talk enough about the positive aspects of growing old. The only thing we should be afraid of is not living the best life we can. Goethe wrote, "An unused life is an early death."

Age doesn't always bring wisdom. Sometimes it brings stupidity. In my own case it's a mixture of both, or perhaps the positive spin is that I've been able to hold on to my puckish, prankish nature even though I now know better. As Lawana Blackwell remarked, "Age is no guarantee of maturity."

Our fear of old age also helps explain the fear of getting sick, and of sickness in others. Illness foreshadows aging. Chronic illness ages you in presidential years. The inevitable decline of the body is sped up, and that frightens people who aren't sick. Mark Twain wrote, "The fear of death follows the fear of life. A man who lives fully is prepared to die at any time." I believe we are never too sick or too old to set another goal.

For the most part, my heath has stabilized, and that enabled me to have a child. By dint of high-tech medical techniques, I am the mother of a smart, funny, beautiful twelve-year-old boy. The only species in which the females live beyond reproductive age are killer whales, pilot whales, and humans. But humans can give birth through surrogate mothers, and I needed a "womb mate" to bring by son into the world.

I was forty-one when Lefty was born. My girlfriends teased me that I could shop for his baby diapers and my adult Depends at the same time. Although when Lefty was teething, my wisdom teeth belatedly erupted—so maybe there's some youth left in the ol' gal yet.

I have always thought of myself as a late bloomer, no matter how old I am. I have developed new life skills in middle age, and I'm still learning new tricks. A human life averages about thirty-five thousand days, and the majority of these days register in the middle to old age range. As Betty Friedan said, "Aging is not lost youth but a new stage of opportunity and strength." Perhaps we late bloomers are just really hardheaded people who never give up trying for what we want out of life. My dad told me that if I had not grown up by the age of fifty, I didn't have to. And I haven't.

OLD PERSON SMELL

If you have a nose, you know there's a particular scent associated with old people. Most people call it "Old Person Smell," but the medical term is nonenal odor. It's a by-product of aging, and according to the *Journal of Investigative Dermatology*, Old Person Smell starts to creep up on you after forty. Britney Spears is just a few years away from smelling like an old lady. Jennifer Lopez has been stinking for years. Is this why they both shill perfumes? The primary cause is the deterioration of the skin's antioxidant defenses. As the skin grows weaker, the natural protective oils in the epidermis oxidize more rapidly. These oxidized chemicals get broken down into tiny stinking molecules called 2-nonenal.

L'EAU DE OLD GEEZER
DECOY PERFUME BOTTLE

Cut out the l'eau de old geezer bottle and tape over
your cheap perfume or cologne.
Now it's disguised!

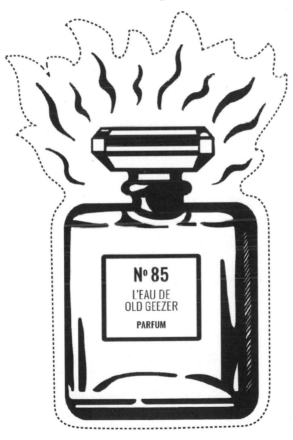

HOCKEY MOM

It took almost two years for my medical team to diagnose my condition as sarcoidosis of the central nervous system. During this phase I went from acutely ill to chronically ill. The acute stage is the emergency, "oh-my-God-am-I-gonna-die?" stage.

I developed a coping strategy to help me endure this time of diagnostic uncertainty. When I went to the corner deli to buy milk, I'd search the dairy case for the milk carton with the longest lead time. My goal was to stay above ground until the date the milk soured. For two years I lived my life from milk carton to milk carton.

When the immediate danger is past and you get into the swing of your new disease, you've matriculated to the chronic phase, where you learn to live with and attempt to manage your serious, unpredictable illness. This is where I am now, and I've been here for a while. A lot has happened to me in the past decade and a half; the best thing was the arrival of my son, Lefty.

It is estimated that 25 percent of women experience fertility issues, and I count myself in this esteemed group. Sarcoidosis, uterine tumors, and the chemotherapy I underwent for both conditions robbed me of my prime baby-making years. My husband and I wanted a child, so we underwent a long process of egg harvesting (well, I did) and implantation (well, my surrogate mom, my womb mate, did) and the result was the handsomest and funniest member of our family.

In our small family, we don't feel like anyone is missing, no matter how many times certain jackasses exclaim, "You only have one? You'd better get going and give him a sibling." Or the helpful "Only children are spoiled and don't get along well with others. We'll pray for you." Well, we're all set, thanks, and I don't think Lefty is spoiled at all. "What if something happens to your son? This is why we have two." Should I get an extra husband, just in case? (Actually, I kind of like that idea.) Usually these uniformed gasbags don't know that the Good Ship Fertility has sailed; I couldn't have more children even if I did want to, no matter how many times a week the guy at the deli tells me I need another kid. Just producing one viable embryo was a major medical achievement. But I'm focused on what we do have, not what we do not. Our family is the perfect size, just the three of us.

I always thought my sisters were crazy when they would tell me that they would not trade one day of being a mother to their kids. Now I get it. My son is now twelve years old, and for the past five years he has been the goalie for a travel hockey team. So far, he's played through the Mites, Squirts, Peewee, and Bantam divisions. The second greatest thing that's happened in the last decade is that my chronic illness is now more manageable. Now, instead of living my life through time measurements dictated by the American Dairy Association, I am counting my longevity by the USA Youth Hockey Age Classifications. I am looking forward to cheering him on as he progresses through the next level.

Hockey is more than a game for us; it's a way of life. It demands a lot from the players and their entire family. I know; I grew up with the game. I am the daughter of a goalie and the mother of a goalie. Perhaps the goalie gene skips a generation? My physical limitations include chronic pain, impaired vision, neuropathy in my hands, and the inability to turn my head to the right. For the past few seasons, I've been wearing a walking cast and sometimes need a cane to get around. If I did have the goalie gene I'd be riding the pine. My hockey days are behind me, and my hockey mom days are ahead of me. But I've learned a lot from watching my son work so hard at his sport, and I've learned to love being a hockey mom.

It's a demanding game, not only for the players but for the player's entire family. If your kid plays soccer, baseball, or basketball, they can go to the backyard or to the park and play in a pick-up game. With hockey, you need ice, so you need scheduled rink time or access to a frozen pond. The players wear nearly double their weight in protective equipment, and they need someone to haul them and their gear to practices, games, and tournaments. It is a hockey mom's role to deliver a child once obstetrically and then deliver them to the rink for the rest of eternity.

Hockey players are dedicated, and they don't give up easily. Neither do their moms. Lefty is challenged on the ice, and my challenge is getting him there. The minutiae of daily life are more taxing when you have the stress of a chronic condition, and I often need to regulate my pain medication around his hockey schedule. I see how hard my son and his team practice to improve their game, and I want to be as dedicated as these kids. They don't make excuses or punk out of early morning practices, and when they get banged around, they shake it off.

When they get tired, they dig deeper. They have to manage their time off the ice so they can give 100 percent on the ice. They inspire me. My son is so passionate about the game. The only thing I love as much as my son loves hockey is my son.

It's a rough, scrappy sport, and it's full of surprises. For example, would it surprise you that the first nut cup (also known as a testicular guard) ever sported in a hockey game was worn in 1873? That the first helmet worn in the NHL was in 1973? That it took a full one hundred years for hockey players to consider protecting their brains was as important as protecting their down below?

My friend and Hockey Hall of Famer Brendan Shanahan was asked if hockey was a hard game. He replied, "Is hockey hard? . . . We need to have the strength of a football player, the stamina of a marathon runner, and the concentration of a brain surgeon. But we need to put this all together, while moving at high speeds on a cold, slippery surface while five guys use sticks to try and kill us. Oh yeah, did I mention that this whole time we're standing on blades an eighth of an inch think? Is ice hockey hard? You tell me."

I'll tell *you* that the sinister vapors emanating from a hockey bag would flatten most people. It's like getting sucker-punched in the face by an invisible roundhouse of adolescent BO. After taking a peek into the closet that houses Lefty's sports gear, my sister Kate remarked, "I don't think the Yankee Candle Company is going to come out with a fragrance called 'Goalie Glove' or 'Winter Seasonal Nut Cup.'"

Luckily, I no longer have a sense of smell; years of chemotherapy and a neurological impairment can knock that right out of your head. Since I can't smell a thing, I am extra-vigilant about cleaning his equipment: skates, pads, gloves, blockers, helmets, and, of course, nut cups. Nobody wants to parent the smelly kid. I don't want his gear to reek.

But the deodorizing sprays you can buy in the laundry aisle don't cut it with Lefty. He didn't want to smell like flowers or a spring meadow. I needed the hard stuff. I went online and found something called Gorilla Wash, which is what zoo-keepers use to hose down their primates. It came in a zoologi-cal size bottle, and I sprayed Lefty's gear generously. I guess I should have read the instructions first, which urged me to "dilute before using." I couldn't smell it, but I could see the stink lines emanating off his jersey, the way Charles Schultz drew the character Pig Pen. The Gorilla Wash, I was informed, smelled even worse than his sweaty socks. I'll stick to soaps and deodorizers meant for humans from now on, although I am sorry I don't get to tell my sisters that I wash my son's gear with zoological products.

Hockey players have many early mornings and for our three-person home team, breakfast is the main meal we share rather than a traditional family dinner. With my husband's professional travel and Lefty's practice and extracurricular activities, we're most likely to be together in the morning. I saw a coffee mug at a tournament that said: "It's a great morn-ing when your kid's face is on the box of Wheaties and your husband's face is on the milk carton." In our society, where even the youngest members of the family leave home early in the morning and sometimes come back late at night, when family dinners are a dim memory like dial telephones and eighteen-hour girdles, breakfasting together is a way to con-vey the sense of parental protection and affection kids need to feel secure and cared for.

I have to take a lot of medication in the morning, and I need something more than black coffee and dry toast; many prescriptions must be taken with food. There is strong evidence that people who don't eat breakfast don't perform as well as people who do. The morning meal supplies energy and nutrients the body needs after its long overnight fast. That's for people who are healthy. It's doubly true for me, challenged as I am by sarcoidosis. I need strength to keep up with my son.

A further incentive is a study of 281 death row inmates, which revealed that only 7.5 percent chose breakfast as their final meal. From this study, I have concluded that breakfast eaters are 92.5 percent less likely to be convicted of serious crimes than those who go without. If this information doesn't inspire you to get your butt out of bed and make Eggs James Bond, I don't know what will.

- -

EGGS JAMES BOND

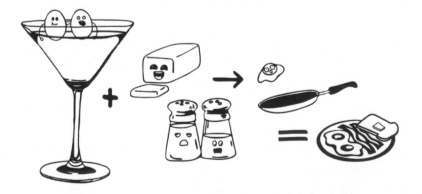

Playing goalie burns a lot of calories, and my skinny string bean son needs two dinners a day to keep up with his nutritional needs—one before practice, and one after. I make the early dinner, and the second one he makes for himself. His favorite meal (and really the only one he knows how to make for himself) is Eggs James Bond. The killer spy ate eggs in just about every book, and in the short story "The Plaza Hotel," author Ian Fleming gives his personal recipe for eggs: Scramble eggs in butter, serve over buttered toast, and pour melted butter over the whole mess. A group of doctors once calculated that if Bond were a real person, he would have died of the three deadly habits—cirrhosis from the shaken martinis, cancer from the smoking, and high cholesterol from the eggs—by the age of fifty-nine. My son doesn't drink or smoke, and I'm hoping that playing hockey will be better for his heart health than assassinating the enemies of the Queen.

- -

Being a hockey mom means spending a lot of time at the rink and long road trips to tournaments. It is in these quieter moments, in between the fanfare of the big victories and the disappointment of losses, where we have shared great memories. The game has brought us closer in a way I never thought a sport ever could. I have physical limitations, so I could not tighten the laces on his skates or adjust his goalie pads. My hands are too weak, and my fine motor control is a bit dodgy. It isn't a big deal, but my son never knew me as a healthy person. My being a hockey mom has helped Lefty understand what I can and cannot do.

I've also experienced profound and unexpected sources of compassion in hockey. One of my kid's teammates asked why he never sees me around the locker room. I explained that I didn't have the dexterity to help Lefty suit up. The kid skated away and came back a few moments later and said, "You seem to have a lot going on and I never want you to worry about your son when he is on the ice. I'm a defenseman and I will always protect our goalie." The kid was twelve years old, but you know what? I don't worry about Lefty out there on the ice.

I want Lefty to have his own experiences, away from my prying eyes. I don't sit in the rink and watch every practice and game. I want him to figure out ways to deal with frustrations and disappointments on his own. I don't see how I'm being useful if I'm all over him like moles on Grandma. He's learning independence and the important skill of being able to tell a great story from his own point of view. And if you play hockey, there's no way to tell a great story without name-dropping the players with the filthiest names of all time:

- Ron Tugnutt—Bruins
- Harry Dick—Blackhawks
- Radek Bonk—Senators
- Bill Quackenbush—Bruins
- Dick Duff—Canadiens
- Grant Clitsome—Red Wings
- Luca Cunti—Tampa Bay Lightning

Through the great game of hockey, Lefty and I have learned the values of nutrition, dedication, determination, and teamwork. He is learning about setting goals as well as scoring them. This is important for him, as he is a goalie and consequently not scoring very much.

When the sticks are slashing and the elbows are flying, you have to be prepared to take the hits. When things are easy, you miss the chance to learn how tough you are. Hockey gives Lefty a chance to prove to himself that he can do it. In hockey, there is a penalty for what's called "embellishment." It's when a player overreacts to an injury during play. The embellishment penalty is a way to call out a faker. My son teases me when I'm having a pain episode: he imitates the expression on my face and my broken bobble head hunched-over posture in order to make me laugh. He has threatened to give me an embellishment penalty if I don't shake it off. It is a reminder to not wallow, that life is going to give you some hits and you have to get up and keep going. I can't call a timeout on being his mom. If Lefty can stand in front of the goal and face a barrage of 90 mph slap shots, I can find a way to suck it up and get him to the rink. It's tough to live as a person with chronic illness, but you know who else is tough? Hockey players.

WILBUR WRIGHT, A HOCKEY FIGHT, A DENTAL MISFORTUNE, AND THE BIRTH OF AVIATION

When Wilbur Wright was eighteen, he was smacked in the puss with a stick while playing pond hockey with friends. His front teeth were knocked out from the hit. (The perpetrator was a neighborhood bully named Oliver Crook Haugh, who went on to be one of Ohio's most notorious murderers. With a middle name like Crook, people really ought to have seen that coming.)

Wilbur's injury wasn't life threatening, but the mutilation affected him deeply. Wilbur had been an athletically and intellectually gifted young man who excelled in school, but after the accident, he became withdrawn and depressed, and he dropped plans to attend Yale University. He spent the next three years as a virtual recluse at his family's home in

Dayton, Ohio. His companions were his father's scientific and mathematical journals.

When Wilbur's brother Orville came back from school, the two brothers capitalized on the national bicycle craze, and they opened a repair and sales shop called the Wright Cycle Exchange. They began manufacturing their own brand of bikes and used the funds from bike sales to pay for Wilbur's growing passion for aviation, culminating in the famous first-ever powered flight at Kitty Hawk. So, a hockey accident is responsible for tiny coach seats, suitcases with broken wheels, and the stewardess trick of "crop dusting" passengers they don't like with intestinal gas. The lesson here: always wear your mouth guard.

- -

HOCKEY MOM COASTERS

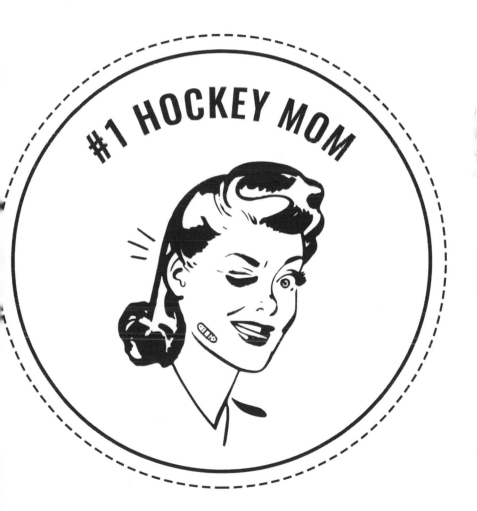

STAGES OF HAGGLING

As MY DOCTOR ONCE said, "We are all temporarily able bodied." My sister Kate suggested that if one day she ever loses a leg, she doesn't want one of those Oscar Pistorius high-tech prosthetic limbs that looks like a rake. "I want an artificial leg," she announced, and went on to describe a 1950s-style wooden leg tapering down to a foot carved in the shape of a clunky old-fashioned shoe and painted brown.

Kate's birthday is two days after Christmas, so I always try to get her exactly what she wants so she doesn't feel cheated out of any gifts. Just recently I hit the jackpot and I found a genuine antique leg prosthesis, just as she described. I can't wait to see the look on her face when she unwraps it.

In the course of my research, I found a Civil War museum that was going out of business and was able to purchase three wooden peg legs. I'm still looking for a fourth because I thought I could make a nice table or standing desk for my husband, though he doesn't share the same enthusiasm for prosthetics that Kate and I do. His last Christmas gift was what's called a "Dorrance appliance," more commonly known as a hook, for someone who's lost a hand. When my husband unwrapped it he was nonplussed. My son looked at me in horror and asked, "Can you please stop giving Dad creepy gifts for Christmas?"

Maybe I will. But I still have an African American male size fifteen left foot in my gift box. Who will I give that to if not John? It's made of silicone and is quite realistic. I wonder about the person I bought it from on eBay . . . what's he doing now? Did he get a new foot? Or was he desperate for money and is just making do without? Maybe I should send it back.

Of course I'm now somewhat disabled myself, though I haven't lost any of my body parts . . . yet. The nerve damage in my left hand has rendered my fingers useless, unable to grasp. At this point they're more decorative than useful. I had to tape the pen to my index finger and thumb just to write this sentence. Although I don't have any artificial limbs, there's been an inevitable process of adjustment to my lessened capabilities. In her research on the terminally ill, Elisabeth Kübler-Ross identified a series of five distinct emotional stages experienced by patients facing the reality of impending death. The Kübler-Ross stages of grief are:

- Denial
- Anger
- Bargaining
- Depression
- Acceptance

When I was confronted with the reality of living the rest of my life in a diminished state, I went through my own series of emotional reactions. I now refer to them, in honor of a friend who is similarly immature, as the Duffy-Gasparini Stages of Haggling:

- Sniveling
- Wallowing
- Finger-pointing
- Whining
- Wondering: how sick do I have to get in order to get one of those little helping hands monkeys?

As with prosthetics, my sister Kate and I have been intrigued by helper animals since childhood, beginning with dogs. In high school, Kate studied up on their history, and informed us all at dinner one day, "The first service animals were guide dogs that assisted German veterans who'd been gassed and blinded in World War I. By 1929, guide dog training had spread to other countries, including the United States. That year Dorothy Harrison Eustis, an American dog breeder, trained a female German shepherd named Buddy for a Nashville resident named Morris Frank. Mr. Frank and Buddy embarked on a publicity tour to convince Americans of the abilities of guide dogs and to allow people with guide dogs access to public transportation, hotels, restaurants, and schools." We were agog.

Inspired by the legacy of Dorothy Harrison Eustis as related by Kate, our little sister Buff raised a puppy for the Seeing Eye foundation. Volunteers care for young pups until they are mature enough to begin training to become a visually impaired person's companion. Buff's dog Gibson was a Golden Labrador Retriever puppy, a hair-raising furball of energy who was inflicted on our family for a year.

Gibson went through a chewing phase that lasted the entirety of his fostering with us. He ate through the stairs of our redwood deck, he gnawed through the bow of our sailboat, and he masticated every non-metal bit of my father's lawnmower.

He chewed through everything except his chew toys. My dad prayed that the visually impaired person who ended up as the human companion to Gibson wouldn't have a wooden leg.

My friend Doris is an ardent supporter of a program called Puppies Behind Bars. When she first mentioned it, I figured this was the place where all the rogue pit bulls and savage ankle-biting dachshunds are penned up after committing their dirty dog deeds. But it's actually a program in which prison inmates foster dogs that will grow up to be companion canines.

Jailbirds have helped raised guide dogs before, but this program expands the idea to service dogs for wounded war veterans, and dogs that work with law enforcement detecting explosives. It's been wildly successful. The prisoners experience the unconditional love of a puppy, and the puppy learns the skills of a working dog. Plus there's very little wood in prison, and I imagine the dogs learn pretty quickly not to chew on the iron bars of the cells.

It made me wonder if prisoners ever train drug-sniffing dogs. What if the positive effect of participating in a dog-raising program just isn't enough to keep a guy from committing more crimes after he gets out? What if he trained the very dog whose incredible nose for the odor of marijuana winds up busting him in the future? Can you imagine the moment the man and the dog lock eyes in recognition, just before the guy gets hauled away in handcuffs? Unbearably sad, right? Doris says this doesn't actually happen, but she doesn't know everything.

I was an animal agnostic, and never knew what I was missing. Three months ago a buddy found a used cocker spaniel on death row at an animal shelter and thought my son would be the perfect human companion for him. We named him

Ravioli, and I'm crazy about this dog. I never knew I had the capacity to love or even like a pet. Now I get why most people love dogs and why there is no one more annoying than a convert. Anatole France wrote that, "Until you have had the love of an animal in your life, part of your soul remains unawakened." Ravioli woke me.*

Oxytocin is the "happiness hormone," which can reduce stress and boost your immune system. It's released during intimate physical contact, such as cuddling a romantic partner or cradling a newborn, which why it's also called the "bonding hormone." Stroking a pet can also cause your body to release oxytocin. Ravioli seems to mainline oxytocin into my wizened corpus. I am besotted, and I spend hours petting him. See? I warned you about converts; we are insufferable.

Ravioli is a sweet companion animal, and my loss of peripheral vision and glaucoma does not yet require a guide dog. The neuropathy in my hands hasn't gotten bad enough to require a helper monkey. Maybe instead of a Seeing Eye dog, I could use a Smelling Nose dog. I've lost my sense of smell, a condition called anosmia, which can happen when you have a neurological impairment or take chemotherapy drugs. But a Smelling Nose dog could be overkill, as a dog's sense of smell is estimated to be ten thousand to one hundred thousand times as acute as a human's. Researchers at Florida State University have compared dogs' sense of smell to humans' visual acuity: if a dog's eyesight was as good as their sense of smell, what humans can see at a third of a mile, a dog could see three thousand miles away. That's like seeing the Hollywood sign from New York City. I don't think I need that kind of surrogate

---

* He was saved through Big Dog Rescue, if you want a place to support.

nose to let me know that my son's hockey gear stinks to high heaven, though.

Surely there's *some* kind of useful animal assistant I'm eligible for? The Americans with Disabilities Act of 1990 defines service animals as any "Guide dog, signal dog or *other animal* trained to provide assistance to an individual with a disability." [Emphasis mine] This law kicked the metaphorical barn door open for a whole menagerie of potential helper animals, if only I could demonstrate the right infirmity . . . and find the right animal.

The Guide Horse Foundation trains miniature horses as assistance animals for people who for one reason or another cannot have a guide dog. In some circumstances, miniature horses are actually better than dogs as guide animals. These tiny equines have a nearly 360-degree field of vision, because they have eyes on the sides of their head and can see in almost total darkness. They're strong and have enormous stamina, so they are a great option for sporty visually impaired people. They're beneficial if the visually impaired human is overweight or less physically capable. Miniature horses are strong enough to pull their handler upright from a sitting position. They can live to be more than fifty years old; guide dogs have a service life of only eight to twelve years. Training a guide dog can cost up to fifty thousand dollars. Training a guide horse can cost about sixty thousand dollars, but since a horse can be in service five times the length of a dog, it's cost-effective to supply blind people with horses. Plus, the horses wear diapers and little sneakers instead of horseshoes.

One major reason a blind person might prefer a horse is religion. I read about a woman who was born with visual impairments and was eligible for a service animal. Her family is devoutly Muslim and in some Muslim sects dogs are considered unclean. Service dogs must live in the house, and certain beliefs don't allow that. Horses don't have the same stigma and also live outside the house in a stable. With the help of her guide horse, this woman was able to travel and attend college.

My takeaway is that this intrepid woman is a much more forgiving person than I am. If I had to do without a helper animal for years and years until someone came up with guide horses, I wouldn't just go to college. I'd go to law school and sue my parents' asses off.

Speaking of asses, not long ago I asked my husband for a pair of American Standard Donkeys. John quickly located a likely couple. "It's remarkably easy to find used jackasses," he commented.

We went to have a look at the pair and immediately fell in love. They were brothers, named Jake and Mason. They were being kept in Tom Joad-like conditions by a little old lady who was no longer able to maintain them in the style to which they had become accustomed. At the time, I didn't know a thing about caring for donkeys, but her biggest concern was that I not spoil them by giving them apples and carrots. I was thinking, lady, I'm not worried about being a helicopter parent to a pair of lovely animals that have brains the size of walnuts.

I'm now a card-carrying member of the American Donkey and Mule Society and the owner of two "rescued" donkeys. I personally hate the word "rescued," unless you actually charged into a burning orphanage to save your current pet. When you announce you have a rescue, you make it all about you and not the animal. My friend Francis tells me there's a plague of cars in Los Angeles with stickers that read, "Who rescued who?" under a big paw print. I don't know, but I do know who's bragging about it.

Helper monkeys, to my mind the gold standard for service animals, can do many things dogs and horses can't. They are trained to assist their human partners in the home. They can scratch itches, reposition limbs, flip buttons and switches on computers, and microwave a Lean Cuisine lasagna. They can perform many tasks that require hands, like perhaps pouring two monkey fingers of tequila over ice. Oh, I would love a little tequila monkey.

They are primarily used to assist quadriplegics and other people with disabilities like spinal cord injuries. Probably the most amazing thing these primates can do is give their human a sponge bath, and that's what sold me on a helper monkey in the first place. Who wouldn't want a monkey sponge bath?

I've heard, though, that the monkeys can be trouble. Everyone knows monkeys will throw their feces. Adolescent ones will get saucy. I think we all know where the term "spank the monkey" comes from. I don't want that. You may disagree.

I believe that for humans, a service animal can fulfill many functions beyond just helping its owner get around. The animal expands the limits of disability. The owner learns to train and care for another living creature, because the dog needs to eat no matter how the owner feels, and the dog's got to go out for a relief walk even when it's raining. It's a symbiotic relationship. The owner is in service to her animal, too.

- -

THERAPY ANIMALS

It's important to note that there are differences between service animals, therapy animals, and emotional support animals. Service animals, as defined by the Americans with Disabilities Act, help their human companions see, hear, or perform tasks they couldn't physically accomplish on their own. They are highly trained and certified. Therapy animals provide affection and comfort to people in institutional settings, such as hospitals, nursing homes, hospices, and in therapy sessions. These therapy animals are trained to socialize and interact with people when they are on duty.

Emotional support animals help their human companions manage the stresses of life and provide comfort. Although there is no standard program to train emotional support animals, many airlines allow them to fly in the main cabin. My agent Peg once remarked that a Screen Actor's Guild card must come with an emotional support animal, because every single actor she knows travels with one.

- -

HE HELPER MONKEY FINGER PUPPET

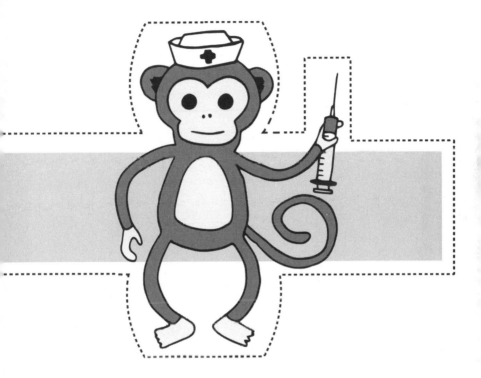

INSTRUCTIONS

1. Cut out.
2. Tape tabs and slip on finger.
3. Presto! This is your 24-hour
private monkey nurse!

EXTRA INNINGS

In almost all of my friendships, I'm the more outgoing of the pair. The exception was Amy. She was from Indiana, and when she arrived in New York, this fresh-faced, corn-fed fashion plate made an impression. Amy was brilliant and bold. She wrote about fashion and culture. We were the same age, yet Amy was more mature, sophisticated, and cosmopolitan. On assignment in Paris she adopted a miniature pinscher she christened Cliché, the name Dorothy Parker—the patron saint of aspiring female writers in New York—gave to her little dog. Compared with Amy, I felt like I just fell off the back of the turnip truck. My family has been rooted in New York City for generations, but she seemed . . . New Yorkier. Some people are just born New York, regardless of the geography of their birth. Amy was born New York.

We met through mutual friends and immediately hit it off. When you join an online dating service, you're matched with a potential partner because you both like the same things. I was drawn to Amy because we both disliked the same things. She hated whining, sentimentality, hypocrisy, the inability to take a joke, and above all dishonorable behavior. I found in her a kindred spirit.

We bonded early through a shared grudge against a fashion editor who'd done each of us a bad turn. I got mad. Amy got that woman's job. She was one of the youngest editors ever hired at the *New York Times*. I always thought of myself as bold, but Amy was bolder.

We also shared bad luck in the health department. Amy and I were struck in the same year with acute illnesses: I had a neurological condition, later identified as sarcoidosis, and Amy was diagnosed with breast cancer. Our hospitals were across the street from each other on the Upper East Side, Amy at Memorial Sloan Kettering and me at New York Hospital/ Cornell Medical Center. We would crank-call each other's rooms and play tricks on our medical teams, such as wearing fake mustaches and false beards during the morning rounds to get a rise out of the interns. We bought remote control fart machines and hid them in each other's rooms to mess with doctors and visitors.

Like good journalists, Amy and I made it our mission to investigate our new surroundings. We'd heard there were secret underground tunnels that heads of state and other dignitaries used to travel between the two hospitals, so we started a competition to see who'd be first to successfully bribe an orderly to wheel her to the VIP catacombs. And we pestered the staff for information about the famous socialite Sunny Von Bulow. She'd been in a persistent vegetative state for decades, and Amy was convinced she could track Sunny down in the warren of high-end suites.

When we got out of the hospital we lived our lives, managing our illnesses, our careers, and our love lives. We both saw the same psychiatrist, who specialized in treating women with serious medical issues. Amy and I both met great guys around this time, and despite the $300-per-hour disapproval of the psychiatrist, we both got married.

Our husbands became friendly, so Amy and her husband came to visit us at our farm in Connecticut. After her health scare, she decided to fulfill her dream of owning a country house too, because why wait? Amy and her husband bought the lake house I had found for them in the next town over, and our friendship grew.

Unfortunately, friendship wasn't the only thing growing. I discovered that I had a blue-ribbon bunch of tumors on my uterus right around the time Amy learned that her cancer had spread to her brain. We found ourselves neighbors once more, though not in the bucolic Connecticut countryside. We were back in the Upper East Side medical complex.

Once again we tried to liven up out hospital stays. We ordered dinner from our favorite restaurants and had it delivered to the hospital. Amy had a manicurist come to do pedicures and manicures. We chatted on the phone and shared movies, magazines, and books.

One of the books we shared was Julia Sweeney's *God Said Ha!*, a touching and hilarious memoir of the time Julia and her brother were both diagnosed with cancer within weeks of each other. Julia had ovarian cancer, and her brother had lymphoma. The Sweeneys teased each other, accusing the sibling of having "Cancer Envy." Julia told him, "You just couldn't stand it, could you . . . me getting all the glory. You couldn't stand it so you got it too, just because you were jealous of the attention." Amy thought I was stealing her thunder by getting another lousy diagnosis the same time she did, for the second time.

We were in our early thirties, and gallows humor helped us through the most frightening procedures. I got a framed portrait of Dr. Kevorkian, aka "Dr. Death," to hang over my bed, and Amy longed for one as well. We'd sneak in liquor and get tipsy, figuring it probably wasn't going to be the booze that killed us. Years later, I saw a contraption called the "Wine Rack," which is a sports bra with a plastic reservoir for smuggling hooch. There's a long tube so you can breast-feed yourself at festivals, concerts, or wherever the mood strikes. Amy would have loved this, and she would have appreciated that it could have saved her thousands of dollars in breast reconstruction.

Amy and I cultivated friendship along with tumors and lesions. We each had surgeries and chemotherapy and psychotherapy. We both kept writing, and we pushed each other to suck it up and not be a pussy about our illnesses. Amy really had no time for pussies. She edited the style section for our nation's paper of record from a hospital bed. She had a caustic edge as a friend, but she was also the most generous and inspiring editor I ever worked for. When *People* magazine voted me onto the worst-dressed list, Amy helped me get the last laugh: she had me write a piece for the *Times* Sunday magazine about how it feels to be categorized as a head-to-toe horror on the worst-dressed list. She knew how to have fun.

Close friends do what's called "mirroring"—they copy each other's behavior. Sometimes this is bad, like when you take up smoking or drink too much because your friends do. And sometimes it's positive. Amy was my badass friend, who dealt with illness like a boss. In mirroring her, I gained the toughness I needed to deal with my rapidly compounding health problems. I like to think Amy mirrored me too, that part of me that that seizes opportunities and flies when the window is open. Maybe I helped Amy decide to go ahead and buy the country house she loved so much.

Amy was one of the wittiest wiseasses I ever met. She was bold and hilarious and cutting. Illness only seemed to egg her on to new heights. We were together at a swanky fundraising dinner for a breast cancer research organization, both of us wearing wigs and scarves to cover up our varying stages of baldness and steroidal puffiness. A model neither of one of us knew very well burst into tears when she saw us. We thought we looked pretty good, considering. This stranger then went in to double-hug us, two people who recoiled from sympathy hugs. After extracting ourselves from her sobbing bosom, I grumbled something under my breath. Amy said in a perfectly normal voice, loud enough for this woman to hear, "Why don't the people who deserve tit cancer get tit cancer, because after that performance, she deserves it!"

Together, Amy and I endured the acute phase of illness. We had the best medical care possible, and it enabled me to transition to the chronic phase. Over a decade later, my chronic phase is ongoing. Amy's is not. She died of metastasizing brain cancer four years after her first diagnosis.

In honor of Amy, I won't be a pussy about it. I'll give you the facts about what happened. It was unbearably sad. Her death really sucked. She died in increments, lost pieces of herself, bit by agonizing bit. First she couldn't hold a pen to edit or write or even scrawl a few words. Her vision went, and she could no longer see the beautiful clothes on which she'd spent her professional life as a groundbreaking fashion critic. Then she lost the ability to speak, to deliver the caustic bon mots that had always delighted me. Then she lost consciousness, and then one day she was dead. I think of her all the time and I really miss her. Cliché the dog died right after Amy; she'd lost too much too.

My story is different. I got sick and stayed sick. I went through the acute phase—the lights flashing, emergency, what-the-hell-happened-to-me stage—and matriculated to the chronic phase. This is where I've been for fifteen years. This is the second phase, where you get accustomed to a whole new life of coexistence with your illness.

But there's more to illness than just a stretch between acute sickness and a dirt nap. Millions of us, people with cancer, lupus, MS, Parkinson's, sarcoidosis, fibromyalgia, Crohn's, cystic fibrosis, and many other diseases will live for years with invisible but persistent illness. Whether it's the miracle of modern medicine or the luck of the draw, we are fated to have to find a way to live for decades with an incurable condition. How about a new name for this stage of life? We've gone beyond chronic into something else. I don't want to make this sound too rosy, because this stage of illness isn't really what you'd call thriving. But it's more than just treading water. I'm not healthy and I never will be, but I'm not hanging by the skin of my teeth either. (What the hell does that even mean, anyway? It's a Bible quote, and unfortunately the author didn't provide a footnote.*)

I read an interview with the former Guns n' Roses bass player Duff McKagan, in which he said that life after getting

---

* The phrase comes from the book of Job, 19:20, and the exact quote is "My bone cleaveth to my skin and to my flesh, I am escaped by the skin of teeth."

sober was like "extra innings"—he'd abused his body so much with drugs and drinking that he "shouldn't be here." And it struck me that that's where I am now, even though I never went wild like my namesake did. I could have croaked, but here I am, playing in extra innings. In extra innings, the game could end suddenly, but you're still getting free baseball.

In the extra innings phase, you can learn from your life and live with vigor and generosity and gratitude. There is a belief that when you lose one sense, the other senses make up for it and become sharper, as in the old wives' tale that a blind person can hear a pin drop across the room. Maybe in extra innings we discover new skills, such as patience and resilience, even as we accept that what we lost won't come back. I've lost my senses of touch and smell and partially my vision, but perhaps my heightened senses of humor and compassion will make up for it? My body is sick, but my spirit is thriving. Maybe in these extra innings we'll call it even?

Extra innings are a bonus. It's a challenge to accept that no matter how well I manage my illness, the symptoms and chronic pain will always be a part of my life. I may mourn for my old life, but now it's up to me to figure out what life I want to lead in extra innings.

When you play sandlot baseball, you flip a coin to see who gets that last time at bat. Flipping a coin goes back to ancient Rome. The head on the coin was the emperor, who was also a living god. If you got the head, god was with you. I won my coin flip. Amy didn't. She was thrown some curve balls, but she gave 110 percent to the very last inning. She was an all-star.

This chapter would have completely struck out with Amy, because another thing she couldn't stand was sports metaphors. I miss her still.

Endometriosis
DREAM DOLL

Mastectomy
DREAM DOLL

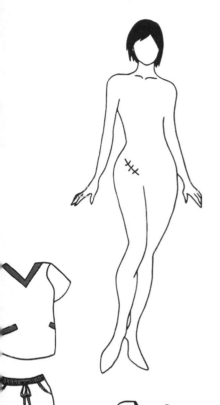

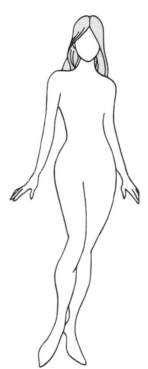

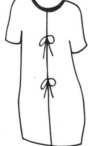

ANTIPELARGIA: THE STORK'S LAW

STORKS LIVE LONG LIVES. They can reach the age of seventy, and when they mate, they mate for life. Younger adult storks feed their elders and offer their extended wings as a crutch to enfeebled parents. Ancient Romans called this loving care of the elderly *antipelargia*. The Roman Senate was so impressed with the stork's generous nature that it passed legislation titled Lex Ciconaria, or the Stork's Law. This law obligated adults to care for their elderly parents "in imitation of the stork."

I may not be quite up to the standard of storks, but I have been working with old folks since I was twelve. I grew up in a conservative Roman Catholic family, and my parents expected their children to find a way to be useful in the world. I volunteered at the local nursing home and enjoyed the one-to-one contact and the challenge of connecting with another soul. In college, I got a degree as a recreational therapist. After graduation, my career and volunteer service was devoted to working with the elderly and disabled populations.

Over sixty-five million Americans care for a chronically ill, disabled, or elderly family member or friend. Nearly 30 percent of the population spends an average of twenty hours per week providing care for their seriously ill loved ones. One of the most difficult and emotionally complicated responsibilities you can take on is caring for an elderly relative. This burden is largely unrecognized. In most cases, family caregivers are not financially compensated, and this enormous domestic workforce is overlooked and undervalued. The economic value of a family or friend caregiver is estimated to be over 500 billion dollars a year—which is about the entire annual budget for Medicare. Many adults are struggling to raise kids while also caring for an ailing relative; they're called the sandwich generation.

The caregiving dynamic is even more complicated when the caregiver is living with a chronic illness of their own. It can feel like you're being crushed by your responsibility to care for someone else while managing your own unpredictable illness. I understand the burden, because I've done it. People like me, with young children, elderly relatives, and a chronic disease, are more like a triple-decker. We have an extra layer—we are the club sandwich generation.

Beyond the unrecognized monetary value of caregiving, the physical and emotional toll of extended domestic healthcare should not be underestimated. Family and friend caregivers are more susceptible to health issues of their own, such as depression, anxiety, and orthopedic injuries. As the primary caregiver, we may be the only person our charge ever speaks to, the only person they see. We can become the receptacle for all their fears and frustrations, a punching bag for their anger. We are often required to perform medically complex tasks that are frightening for both the patient and caregiver. We clean, bathe, cook, do laundry, and tend to their most intimate personal needs. We are the primary social outlet for the patient. It can be crushing. Self-care for the caretaker is not selfish—it's soul-saving. Hospitals and community centers offer support groups and services for caregivers, and it is desperately needed.

Here's the jig. We can all expect that at some point we will either fall ill and need a caregiver, or we will become a caregiver for someone who's ill or injured. We may be called to mother our mother, or become skillful in fathering our father. For fifteen years, my family faced the challenge of caring for my husband's grandmother. My father-in-law died in an accident, and our family inherited the responsibility of caring for his nonagenarian Greek-American mother, Athena. Like most catastrophes, it happened suddenly, with a series of minor catastrophes unfolding one after another in its wake. I thought I had the skill set to deal with being one of the primary caretakers of a cranky, bereft old woman. I don't think an entire mustering of storks would have been able to peck away at her hostility.

Athena's husband died at the age of 103, a year before the unexpected death of her only child. The double blow of losing the two most important people in her life did not blunt her sharp tongue. Sadness and misery were her whetstones, and every indignity, whether real or imagined, honed her ability to cut ever deeper.

When I worked at group homes, nursing homes, and hospice units, I would seek out the grouchy, smelly people. All the sweet old ladies in pink cardigans and blue-tinted curls got the smiles from the staff. I thought the grumpy ones could use the attention too. The difference was that I could leave the nursing home after my shift. But when you have a depressive, angry elder relative in your care, you can't escape. You can't walk away. I had to develop an even thicker skin, selective deafness, and strategic mutism, and summon all my strength even when I had little to spare.

Athena was family, and it was our duty to help care for her. We brought her groceries. We took her to the doctor, hairdresser, and the department store. We'd take her to the family farm in Connecticut for the weekend. I'd call her the first thing in the morning and the last thing at night. We tried our best to help ease the pain of outliving her only child, but we didn't make a dent in her depression.

Once I was watching TV with her, and a commercial came on featuring a series of children declaring, "I was born to be an astronaut," "I was born to be a fireman," and so on. And Athena, who was on the floor doing sit-ups, turned to me and said, "I was born to suffer."

She was born (suffering, one presumes) in a rural Greek village. Yet she carried herself with all the vanity and snobbery of a grand dowager. She flaunted her razor-thin figure. Her speedy metabolism and her tiny waist were a source of eternal pride; she ate like a bird. She executed sets of crunches and marched in place. She was committed to her daily fitness regime. She viewed adipose tissue as a character flaw. I was still modeling, and when she saw me on the cover of a health and fitness magazine, her comment was "You aren't really that big, are you?" I could take it, but she gave her unsolicited opinion on Body Mass Index to her nurses, Bloomingdales' sales associates, her infant great-grandson, and anyone ordering rice pudding in the neighborhood coffee shop. Athena taunted a visiting nurse about her weight so viciously that the poor woman was reduced to tears. The nurse left before the teakettle boiled.

Athena used her cane to nudge shop assistants to hurry them up. I'd double-tip any cab driver that ferried us around the city to compensate for her grousing and fussing. Andy Rooney once said, "The best classroom in the world is at the feet of an elderly person." What I witnessed at the feet of this particular elderly person, besides bunions and hammertoes, was her iron will, her deep faith, and her unshakeable conviction that she was always right.

Athena was no breadstick-boned husk of a woman. She was vital and bossy and unsentimental. She was surprisingly healthy for a wafer-thin centenarian. She had a pacemaker, and after ten years of service, the batteries need to be replaced. We asked if the surgeon could just remove the pacemaker instead. It seemed to keep her kicking, and this was not a woman who was enjoying life. But the cardiologist said it didn't work that way.

The night before she was to get the new battery implanted in her ticker, I slept at her apartment. I had just interviewed the Rolling Stones for an HBO concert special. I made us Kahlua and milk cocktails, and we watched the program. She didn't think my outfit did me any favors, and she helpfully pointed out that the camera adds at least ten pounds. She was fascinated that the Stones had an elderly Greek woman playing guitar. She was referring to Ron Wood.

Before we went to sleep, I told her I loved her and that tonight would be a great night to "go to the light." I was right there in the twin bed next to her, so she need not be afraid. I would be with her and she could end her unhappiness. No neighbor would have to call and report an alarming smell coming from apartment 12P, and this was as good a time as any.

The next morning, she growled from her bed, "I'm still alive."

In her late nineties, she was hit by a car while crossing the street. The only thing that broke was her cane. But she was infuriated that her crisp blue blazer was torn, and raged the entire way to the hospital about her jacket. In the emergency room, I had to fill out medical history and insurance forms. I asked her for her date of birth, and she barked that it was none of my business. I explained that I was not being nosy, but the hospital staff needed to know. "Well," she sneered, "tell them they can ask my mother. She was there when I was born." At that point, her mother had been dead for at least eight decades. Athena was cagey about her age and always excused her vagueness by saying that in Greece all the records were destroyed in World War II. That would have been a valid excuse, except that she and her records had immigrated to the US in the 1920s, right after World War I.

When Athena was ninety-nine, she had a small stroke. Damage to the brain caused by a lack of blood flow is called a "stroke" because in the seventeenth century, it was believed the sufferer was actually "struck by the hand of God." God didn't hit Athena nearly as hard as He might have, but as Athena recovered in the hospital, we realized it was time for other measures. She could no longer live independently and terrorize shopkeepers, doormen, and anyone wearing stretch pants in public. She was nearly a century old, and we had to find an assisted living community. The Greek Orthodox Home for the Aged rejected her for being too old. She hated the swanky Catholic nursing facility just a few blocks away from her Upper East Side apartment. She said it was intolerable because of all the Irish. Of course, I'm Irish Catholic.

We visited a succession of what former poet laureate Donald Hall called "old-folks storage bins" and "for-profit-making expiration dormitories." We finally found a lovely location near our farm in Connecticut. But even though her venue had changed, Athena didn't. Age had not mellowed her, infirmity did not calm her. Her snobbery and ill temper didn't win her any popularity contests with the staff or the residents. She chose to eat every meal alone. If I ever said hello to anyone in the dining room besides her, she'd shout insults at us across the room. The staff served ice cream and pie, and she served stink eye.

The average stay in an assisted living facility is about eighteen months. Athena, as always determined to prove she knew better, doubled that. One December day, I dropped by to send out her Christmas cards. She was in a sour mood; she cranked up the grouchy to eleven for the holiday season. She asked what would happen if she stopped taking her medication. Her nurse said she would die. This answer seemed satisfactory, and from that moment on she refused to swallow her pills. The doctor said it would take about two weeks, and in fact, I could have set my watch by his prediction.

I was familiar with the nursing home rule of thumb that patients are more likely to die around the holidays. The most popular day of the year to die is New Year's Day. On New Year's Eve, the nursing home told us it was time for hospice care. On the drive over, I stopped off at the liquor store and bought several airline-size bottles of Bailey's Irish Cream and Kahlua. I had hoped we could have one last toast together, but by the time I got there, she was very weak and had her eyes closed. I sat with Athena and told her she was loved and had nothing to fear. From working in nursing homes, I'd learned that hearing is the last sense to go. Don't say anything you would not want your loved one to hear. Don't fight over the jewelry or their gold teeth while they are still in the room. Even though it was my last chance to let her have it, I talked about her faith instead.

I took her hand to say good-bye. She opened her eyes and she seemed to perk up. It was like a sleeping tiger had been roused. She tried to bend my fingers backwards; I think she was trying to break them. When she wasn't successful, she extended my middle digit so I was giving myself the finger

I'll never forget her last words. "You stink on ice," she growled. I withdrew my hand and bade a fond farewell. She died that evening, New Year's Eve.

The next morning, my son joined my husband and me in our living room as we made the funeral arrangements with the undertaker. He asked our son, "Would you like to write a letter or make a drawing for your great-grandmother?" Lefty gently reminded him that she had died the night before and he didn't think she would get the note.

The undertaker told us that in our village, in the Berkshire Mountains of northwest Connecticut, the snow and frozen ground made it impossible to bury anyone in the cemetery until the spring thaw. This was news to me. You can put a man on the moon in the cold of space, but you can't put a ninety-pound woman six feet under when the temperature dips below freezing? I asked where she'd be kept until she could be buried. He told me she would be in the basement of the funeral home in the deep freeze. I guess she was stinking on ice, too.

To call her stubborn would be an insult to all other stubborn people. But in the end she had no power to unnerve me. She was a very difficult woman, but I admired her for her toughness. I hope I'm as strong when I get to be her age. She wore hot-pink sequined high tops instead of orthopedic shoes. She was fearless and had driven an ambulance in World War II. She was *sui generis*, one of a kind.

I remember once, near the end of her life, Athena told me that in her mind she was still a nineteen-year-old girl, coming to America to get married. In all the time I spent with her, it was the most beautiful thing she ever said. So that's what I choose to remember of her, the hopeful young girl I never got a chance to meet in person.

- -

TOP FIVE REGRETS OF THE DYING

I've worked at a nursing home. I've interned as a hospital chaplain. I've been at the bedside of dying loved ones and dying strangers, and if there's one thing I'm sure of it's that you don't want regrets to be the last thing on your mind. Caregiver Bronnie Ware has gathered together her observations of the dying in a book called *The Top Five Regrets of the Dying*. As witnessed by Ms. Ware, they are:

1. I wish I hadn't worked so hard
2. I wish I had the courage to express my feelings
3. I wish I had stayed in touch with my friends
4. I wish I'd let myself be happier
5. I wish I had the courage to live my true life, not the life others expected of me

In my experience, most people regret the things they didn't do, such as not taking a vacation, not trying to heal broken relationships, and not saying "I'm sorry" or "thank you" or "I love you" as much as they should have. These regrets always seem doable—I never heard anyone say "I regret not going over Niagara Falls in a barrel." I've also noticed that at the end of life, people often talk to me about their childhood pets or the taste of pastrami on rye. It's the little things that we carry with us, the small, beautiful things we miss when we're dying.

- -

Please!
DO NOT DISTURB

I need my ten minutes

ENTER AT YOUR OWN RISK

THE FLANEUR

IN *Midnight Cowboy*, WHICH won the Academy Award for best picture, one of the most iconic scenes in the film occurs when Dustin Hoffman's character Ratso Rizzo, a pimp, offers to help Jon Voight's Joe Buck become a gigolo. As they cross the street, deep in conversation, a taxi squeals to a stop within inches of them. Ratso bangs on the hood and shouts at the driver.

This wasn't planned. The traffic light changed during the shot, and a real New York City cab drove through the intersection where they were filming. You can hear that Hoffman dropped Ratso's nasal accent and yelled in his own voice, "I'm walking here!" It's now one of the most famous lines in movie history.

I walk the streets of New York myself, dodging cabs as necessary, and I don't mind admitting that those stirring words, uttered by a fictional filthy consumptive gimping pimp, now help impart some pep to my step.

It isn't easy staying fit when you live with chronic health issues. Illness can be an incubator for excuses—and it is a pretty good excuse. But you have to be disciplined enough to dismiss the temptation to recuse yourself from daily exercise.

You need to make every effort to stay as physically fit as possible, especially when you face serious health issues. As my father likes to say, "If you don't take care of your body, where are you going to live?"

I plan on living in this well-used and well-loved body for a good long time, but finding and committing to an exercise plan that worked for me on good days as well as bad was a challenge. I needed to do something to stay fit, but I couldn't tolerate a lot of bouncing around, so aerobics was out. Pilates with sweaty strangers was as torturous as my illness. Weight training dragged me down.

In an effort to help get me moving, my son tied a marshmallow to a toy drone. He'd fly it around the house and have me chase it. I'd call this training method a draw, as I ate the marshmallow once I caught it.

Yoga was a whole separate level of hell, and not only because of all the farting. I don't know how many yogis tried to tell me that the pain was all in my mind. "It's actually in my spinal cord," I'd reply, on my way out of the door. The classes I did get through were always spoiled at the end. The last thing you do in a yoga class is lie flat on your back in the pose called sivasana, or corpse pose, where you're supposed to focus on your breathing. But it seemed that just about every yoga studio in Manhattan plays Jeff Buckley's beautiful and haunting version of Leonard Cohen's "Hallelujah" at the end. I couldn't concentrate on my own breath when I was thinking about Buckley's last gasps in the Wolf River. The other popular sivasana soundtrack was Andrea Bocelli singing "Amazing Grace." First of all, it bothered me when he sang the line "I was blind, but now I see," because, you know, he still is, and he can't. Second, you might know that the hymn was written by

John Newton. He composed this plea for mercy when he sailed into a violent tempest on the Atlantic Ocean on his slave ship. He was a slave trader. Newton was saved, and yet he continued buying and selling humans for years after he composed that little ditty. Maybe you're different, but I found myself unable to empty my mind of all thought when being serenaded by a slave trader's theme song.

AMAZING GRACE

Whit Crane, the lead singer of the metal band Ugly Kid Joe, is a one-man conga line of fun. We dated for several years, he's charming and a total sweetheart, and we remain devoted friends. I went to see him once at Ozzfest, and during sound check he suddenly broke into a rendition of "Amazing Grace." Whit doesn't go for a lot of fancy book learning, so instead of singing "saved a wretch like me," he went with "saved a wench like me." I remember all the roadies stopped working and the techs perked up, and everyone got this look on their face like it was some kind of prayer for racial harmony, instead of a desperate plea to stay alive and sell more slaves. I cannot believe the run that this malevolent little number has had, with some performers having made it their signature. Here are the ten worst offenders:

1. **Mahalia Jackson.** The Queen of Gospel. A legend. Did she know the backstory? I hope not.
2. **Judy Collins.** The folksinger and activist had made a career out of "Amazing Grace," including a version with the Harlem Boys Choir.

3. **Aretha Franklin.** Why? Why?
4. (tie) **Mormon Tabernacle Choir** and **Soweto Gospel Choir.** No, just no.
6. **Elvis Presley.** First he entirely appropriates black culture, and then this.
7. **The Royal Scots Dragoon Guards.** Most probably did not know what the hymn was about.
8. **Mumford and Sons.** Definitely did not know what it was about.
9. **Andrea Bocelli.** Or the yoga-ruiner, as I call him.
10. **Whitfield Crane.** Goes without saying.

- -

I found myself trying to explain to every trainer or class leader that I wasn't interested in getting skinny. My goal isn't to get teeny-tiny or grow major biceps. That ship has sailed, and I've learned to love my chub. I just want to do the best with what I have. I wasn't interested in fitness as a lifestyle, and I'm still not. Some people crave a runner's high; I run from it. But walking? Now that, I can do.

Isaac Newton's first law of motion, also called the Newtonian Law of Inertia, states that an object at rest stays at rest, and an object in motion stays in motion. This means that the natural tendency for things is to keep doing what they're doing. If what you're doing is wallowing on the couch, you'll stay there with your butt softened by a sofa cushion . . . unless a force acts on you. That force can be your own will to make a change.

The Law of Inertia also says that all objects resist change in their state of motion. Meaning it's not going to be easy to break your ass-expanding La-Z-Boy habit. But you've got to try. You've already got some kind of illness, that's bad enough. But a sedentary lifestyle is the greatest single cause of serious health issues. The American Cancer Society followed more than 100,000 subjects, and the study proved that sitting around all day causes a multitude of problems, including premature death. The only way to reverse the problems caused by all the sitting is to get up off your keister and get moving.

I know, you're in pain and you don't feel up to it. I understand, I really do. Perambulation is what our bodies are designed to do, and when that basic activity hurts, it's disheartening. The ability to walk without pain is a gift that we don't have anymore. Being able to walk with pain and not give up is a superpower. It's hard. But no one said being a superhero was easy. Without exercise you will lose even more strength, and you will end up with the muscle tone of a raw clam. Constant inactivity will make your overall health even worse. But it is inspiring that even moderate exercise, such as walking and stretching, will stimulate the release of endorphins, your body's natural painkillers and mood enhancers.

Newton's Second Law says that when a force acts to accelerate a mass, the greater the mass of the object to be moved, the greater amount of force is needed. So the longer you sit there, a pile of human gridlock, the harder it's going to be to get started. But there's an upside—remember the first law: an object in motion stays in motion. It's going to take more energy to haul your carcass up off your needlepoint whoopee cushion that it will to take the first step and every step after that.

Newton's Third Law is that for every action, there is a reaction. What that means for you is that once you get moving, your health will improve. Small changes will make a big difference. You don't have to run a marathon. Just move. Don't get marooned on your recliner. Get up and leave the butt-shaped dent in front of the screen, get outside, and start walking. Your body and mind and overall health will improve. I guarantee that if you don't see results, I will refund to you any change I can find in your couch cushions.

Once you start walking, the Newtonian Law of Inertia becomes your friend. A body in motion will stay in motion. Daily walks will become habitual. Psychologists have found that a habit maintained for three weeks can become a habit for a lifetime. Habitual actions create new neural pathways in your brain—so in just twenty-one days, you can literally rewire your brain for daily walks. If you're looking for a way to boost your mood and deflate your spare tire, the solution is right at your feet.

When you get moving, everything changes, physically and psychologically. Our bodies are optimized for walking by millions of years of evolution, so you've got that going for you. Walking is more than perambulation between two destinations. Just thirty minutes of walking each day can improve your health and reduce the risk of heart attack, diabetes, and stroke. Again, I'm not talking about getting ripped—all I want is for you to get out and walk around the block. But when you add it all up, the average person in their lifetime walks the equivalent of traveling around the world, TWICE! (I know that many people reading this are physically unable to walk, and I don't mean to leave you out. Please see the sidebar for some other ideas.)

ADAPTIVE EXERCISE

I profoundly enjoyed my teenage volunteer experience in the nursing home, so in college I studied recreational therapy and then worked as professional in the field. As a Recreational Therapist Emeritus, I know that the goal of any adaptive activity is to maximize ability and focus on what you can do. As I never tire of saying, it is a mistake to do nothing just because you can only do a little. Some days I am in bed because of intense nerve jangling pain and I can't even walk around my apartment. When I'm hopped up on goofballs and look like Gomer Pyle in a gas leak, I squeeze therapy balls with my hands and do very light exercises. I make circles with my ankles and wrists. It's not Bikini Booty Boot Camp; I just want to keep the blood circulating and engage those of my muscles that are not quivering in pain.

It takes energy to live. You burn 1.5 calories per minute just lying still while your body performs its basic functions, such as pumping blood and farting. When you go from lying down to sitting up, you burn 25 percent more calories—that's 1.875 calories a minute!

So sit up. And when the pain flare passes, get moving. Get up from your chair and stretch once in a while. Work standing up if you can. Walk to the store, or just to the corner, or shake your keister around the house to Beyoncé. It all helps.

Adaptive exercise is a category of physical activities tailored for people with physical limits, such as severe pain, paraplegia, or anything that might make my walking plan hard to put into action. The National Center on Health, Physical Activity, and Disability has a wealth of resources to help you find an activity that works for your situation; they're at http://www.nchpad.org. The National Multiple Sclerosis Society is another good place to try. Its website is http://www.nationalmssociety.org. And don't assume that your physical condition mean that all you can do is little ankle circles like me. Lindsay Hilton was born without arms or legs, but plays rugby anyway: https://www.youtube.com/watch?v=uPOcM5BH-hU. And via the NCHPAD, quadruple amputee Bob Lujano demonstrates how he does interval training:

https://www.youtube.com/watch?v=ysrV0zhcMmI.

New research has shown that just watching other people exercise can have an actual physical benefit. This is good news for me, because on some days my exercise program consists of watching videos of Rodney Yee in his Speedo doing yoga on the beach.

- -

We are a nation of housecats. Most people in developed countries sit on their keisters all day at their jobs and then at home in front of a screen. 97 percent of our time is spent indoors. It's not good for you, and pedaling on a bike to nowhere for an hour isn't going to make up for ten or twelve hours sitting on your caboose. It's far more effective to integrate movement throughout the day instead. Take a fifteen-minute break and walk around the block—you'll come back refreshed and more productive, too. Dr. Muir Gray, a leading public health advocate in the UK, believes that Type 2 diabetes should be renamed "walking deficiency syndrome," because the disease can be a result of our sedentary lifestyles and modern environment.

People who do moderate exercise such as walking (or golf, swimming, or dancing) describe feeling more energetic, more socially connected, and more emotionally balanced. They also report decreased pain and depression. Walking reduces stress, blood pressure, and body fat. Just carrying around extra body fat can impact pain symptoms. Even an additional five to ten pounds can increase the stress on your knee and hip joints. Weight management and incorporating any exercise plan are often overlooked complements to pain management. Walking also improves quality of sleep, strengthens the heart, and increases muscle and bone strength. Unlike a stationary bicycle or a treadmill, it takes you places. Hey, you might even find some money on the street!

The benefits of walking aren't exactly news, either. Over two hundred years ago, Thomas Jefferson not only informed us that we had been endowed by our creator with the rights to life, liberty, and the pursuit of happiness, he urged us out of the house with these words: "Walking is the best possible exercise. Habituate yourself to walk very far." And Charles Dickens, who was not really paid by the word but wrote as if he were, said, "The sum of the whole is this; walk to be happy; walk to be healthy. The best way to lengthen our days is to walk steadily and with a purpose. The wandering man knows of certain ancients, far gone in years, who have staved off infirmities and dissolution by earnest walking—hale fellows, close up on ninety, but brisk as boys."

Well, you want to be brisk as a boy at ninety, don't you? I do, and I'm a woman. Rene Descartes described the present as what divides your past from your future. The disease that's keeping you holed up in the house began in your past, but your future is yours, so start moving in the present.

I find that a pedometer helps get me going. It's incredibly satisfying to look and see the number of steps going up, up, up. Counting steps can be addictive, and by setting goals you'll find yourself increasing movement in your daily life. Ten thousand steps a day is a common target, though that's for an able-bodied person; your goal may be different. My family is competitive, and we all have pedometers, so if I don't make my personal goal by the end of the day, I'll march around my apartment in my knickers, pacing like a Silverback Gorilla until I hit my target number. My husband says bouncing my knees while I'm sitting on my butt drinking a glass of wine doesn't count, but my pedometer doesn't know that.

One related health tip I can share is to not wear a candy bracelet on the same wrist as your pedometer. You can crack a tooth if you latch on to the wrong item.

- -

WHY TEN THOUSAND STEPS?

The origin of idea that you should walk ten thousand steps a day comes from a Japanese brand of pedometer marketed as the "manpo-kei," which translates to "the ten thousand steps meter." The idea of walking ten thousand steps a day became accepted as a goal, but the American Centers for Disease Control actually recommends a minimum of eight thousand steps per day.

- -

Walking is not just a physical exercise; it's a metaphysical exercise as well. There's a transformative power in perambulation. Walking engages not only our bodies but also our minds. As Friedrich Nietzsche wrote, "All truly great things are conceived by walking."

Flaneur is the French word for walker, or saunterer. A flaneur is someone who walks as a mode of self-expression and exploration. For the flaneur, walking is not about getting from point A to point B, or about getting in shape. The act of walking is its own reward. A flaneur walks the city in order to experience it, to fully participate through observation and peregrination.

The original flaneurs were literary types in nineteenth-century Paris. They were connoisseurs of the streets. Poet Charles Baudelaire, a noted flaneur, called himself a "botanist of the sidewalk." Flaneurs transformed what was mindless transit into mindful exploration. They walked to become calmer, more insightful and meditative, in the belief that the quality of thoughts that erupt during walks are superior to less ambulatory thinking. Flaneurs would sometimes walk a pet turtle or lobster on a leash, just to enforce a leisurely, contemplative pace.

Medical researchers report that walking stimulates the brain and enhances creativity because the rhythmic circumambulation reflects the cadence of our thoughts. Every step propels us through space, but also propels our thoughts. The visual stimulus of the panorama unfolding before us introduces new inspiration and creates new ideas. Walking provides an opportunity to process the day; it is a form of contemplation. It engages and connects you with your environment, and though you may walk alone, you are not lonely. Honore de Balzac wrote that flaneurie, the act of flaneuring, is "the gastronomy of the eyes." Each step satisfies our hunger for experience and knowledge. In walking, Baudelaire said, "The flaneur is capable of finding a remedy for the ever-threatening ennui."

Some of the greatest minds in history were flaneurs. Beethoven composed music in his head during his daily walks.

Aristotle's school of thought was named the Peripatetic school, because he believed that philosophical ideas were best explored in *peripateu*—while strolling about. Einstein, Darwin, Tchaikovsky, Thoreau, Dickens, Whitman, Goethe, and Steve Jobs all enjoyed their mind-expanding daily constitutionals (though not at the same time).

A flaneur is always a man, but only because a woman is called a flaneuse. The American transcendentalist and feminist Margaret Fuller was a flaneuse, a deep thinker and long walker, often in the company of her transcendentalist friends Emerson and Thoreau. Novelist Frances Trollope was a flaneuse, as was her French contemporary George Sand.

I was immediately drawn to the idea of a leisurely stroll around the city, because as much as I love walking around town, I'm never going to take the gold medal in speed walking. I find flaneuring an effective remedy for my chronic pain, and, so far, it has kept the ever-threatening ennui at bay. I enjoy the fertile solitude of an evening walk. My neurologist says that walking is actually a self-medicating behavior, because repetitive motions such as walking can have the same effect on the brain as meditation. Walking can calm the mind, distract it from chronic pain, steer it away from intrusive or destructive thoughts. The pattern of one foot following the other allows the brain to return to the motion.

Our human brains and bodies were created to do our best thinking while in motion. Human thought is connected to movement, and movement to a healthy brain. The amygdalae are two small parts of your brain, one in the prefrontal cortex of each hemisphere. They're the size and shape of almonds—*amygdala* is Greek for almond. Despite their small size, the amygdalae play a crucial role in how we understand emotions and relate to others. People with a large social circle tend to have large amygdalae. It's the amygdalae that create neurochemicals that act as natural pain relievers when we are engaged in self-soothing activities, like walking.

The hippocampus is a structure in the brain that is crucial to the formation of memories. Even in healthy people it begins to atrophy in your mid-fifties. But psychologists have discovered that the hippocampus can be expanded by habitual walking, and neurologists agree that walking can increase memory in old age. So remember to walk, don't forget!

Exercise such as walking is believed to be as effective as anti-depressants in elevating your mood. So begin a walking routine for your heart and your head. Your new career as a flaneur will unlock the capacity to positively change other habits for the better. Make your motto "solvitur ambulando," which in Latin means "it is solved by walking."

Studies show that walking in a natural setting, such as a park, can reduce brain fatigue and decrease the risk of dementia. But more than half of the world's population now lives in cities, surrounded by asphalt jungles. I love New York, and I get a tremendous amount of happiness walking its dirty streets, filthy sidewalks, and stinking alleys. In cities, we've largely cut ourselves off from the restorative power of nature.

Shinrin-yoku is a practice that can be translated from Japanese as "forest bathing." Developed in the 1980s, it is a pillar of preventive health care and healing in Japan, and it consists simply of walking in nature. Japan's Minister of Health has prescribed a weekly dose of shinrin-yoku for every citizen. The exposure to nature calms the central nervous system and stimulates physical health. In the US, we sunbathe, lying motionless on a beach towel absorbing cancer-causing radiation. In

Japan, a forest bath increases metabolic and aerobic fitness and decreases stress, anger, anxiety, and depression.

Shinrin-yoku, walking in nature, makes intuitive sense because trees are powerful symbols in almost every culture. For all of human history, our ancestors relied on trees. They were a source of shelter, food, protection, medicine, fire, and weapons. The growth of trees, their strong but flexible branches, the annual bearing of fruit and its subsequent decay, and the revival of their foliage in spring are powerful symbols of life, death, and resurrection. The veneration of trees is known as dendrolatry, and this worship is linked to the ideas of fertility, growth, mortality, and rebirth. A recent study revealed that if your hospital room has a view of trees, rather than the parking lot, you can actually heal more quickly.

My husband's family has a working farm in Connecticut, and though I'm a city girl I've come to appreciate the power of trees. We have apple orchards and maples we tap for syrup. My husband planted a collection of pear, peach, and cherry trees he calls the Fruit Cup. I now practice my own form of shinrin-yoku in addition to flaneuring my way around New York. I'm still adhering to my medical regime of morphine and steroids, but wherever I am I'll take a walk as part of my daily prescription for pain relief, general good health, mental inspiration, and simple enjoyment of my surroundings.

- -

WALKING INTO HISTORY

Edward Payson Weston was a champion of walking as a means to fitness, and his marathon walks from city to city were the marvel of the nineteenth-century United States. He was America's most famous pedestrian. His first step as a notable walker was when he lost a bet over the 1860 presidential election and had to walk from Boston to Washington, DC. It took him ten days, and he slogged through snow, rain, ice, and mud. He arrived in Washington at five p.m., and walked straight into Abraham Lincoln's inaugural ball.

In 1909, on his seventieth birthday, he began a walk from New York City to San Francisco. Weston wanted to grab the spotlight back from the emerging sport of running, but also to prove that his vigorous lifestyle had kept him strong. It took him 105 days to cross the continent, plagued by wind and snow in the Rockies and searing heat in the Nevada desert. Dissatisfied with his performance, the next year he walked back in just seventy-six days. Sadly, Weston was hit by a taxi at the intersection of 7th Avenue and West 11th Street in 1927 at the age of eighty-eight, and he never walked again. (Decades later, my dad was walking home from school and was hit by a car at the exact same intersection, though he was neither permanently crippled nor a champion walker.)

- -

YOU'RE #1 TROPHY

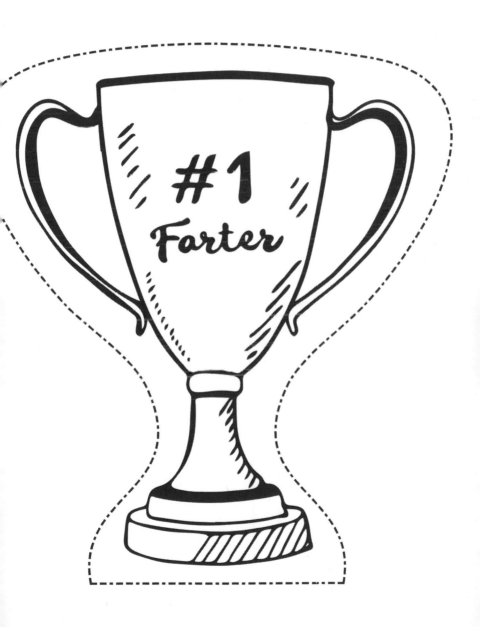

WISE GUYS

I TREASURE THE MEMORIES of the summers I spent in a scrappy shared beach house on Shelter Island, off the east coast of Long Island. I was past the worst of my acute phase of sarcoidosis, but I was only tentatively emerging into a more active life. Shelter Island is bucolic and quiet, and it can be reached only by ferry. It was the perfect place for me. I was lucky to be able to share a crowded beach shack with good friends as I recovered my strength and my spirit.

My friend Mary, who was visiting for the weekend, was talking about an archeological dig she was going to participate in—not in the deserts of Egypt, but at the historic Sylvester Manor on Shelter Island, within easy walking distance from our house. It still belonged to the family who'd built it one hundred years before the Revolution.

"Why don't you come?" she said. "You'll have fun. You're nosy, you like going through other people's stuff."

"I don't know if I'm up for digging trenches yet. I'm not too far from needing a six-foot trench myself."

"This will be easy. It's poking through the old kitchen trash heap looking for broken pottery."

"Well, since you make it sound so attractive, I'll give it a try."

I tagged along with Mary, and before we got our hands dirty looking for centuries-old chicken bones and rusty nails, we were given a tour of the home and grounds. The grande dame of the manor, Alice Fiske, led us through a formal garden that was populated by large marble busts. One particular curly head caught my eye, and I asked who he was when he wasn't dead.

"Oh, that's Marcus Aurelius," Mary said off-handedly.

If she could identify a Roman Emperor who'd been dead for thousands of years just by his profile, I knew I'd better step up my classical studies game. I dove into reading about Ancient Greece and Rome, and brushed up on Stoic philosophy.

Philosophy translates to "love of wisdom." That's something we all share with Zeno of Citium, the founder of Stoicism. He chose to teach his ideas not in a school, shut away from the public, or in a cave, like Plato. He taught from a porch, or stoa, where anyone could hear him. Zeno's main idea was that humans cannot control what happens to us; we can only control how we react to it. His teachings spread widely, and the Roman Emperor Marcus Aurelius, later immortalized in that curly-headed bust, was one of many who continued the philosophical tradition of the Stoics.

- -

PLATO

Just a few words about the Greek philosopher Plato. It just doesn't seem fair that Plato is most commonly known as a descriptor used to emphasize that a relationship between two people is not sexual, it is a meeting of the minds, not the commingling of sexy parts. Here are three Platonic facts and three great quotes so you'll know him as more than just a euphemism for not porking:

- Plato was his nickname; his actual name was Aristocles. The nickname "Plato," meaning broad, was given to him because of his broad shoulders.
- He was a student of Socrates.
- Aristotle was one of Plato's pupils.

Three Memorable Quotes Attributed to Plato

- "One of the penalties for refusing to participate in politics is that you end up being governed by your inferiors."
- "Be kind, for everyone you meet is fighting a hard battle."
- "You can discover more about a person in an hour of play than in a year of conversation."

- -

I went on to read other Stoics such as Epictetus, who wrote "The Art of Living." Epictetus was born a slave in the Roman Empire around AD 55. His master was one of Emperor Nero's administrators, and like Nero he was cruel. Epictetus was beaten so severely that his leg was broken, resulting in a permanent disability and chronic pain. He persevered through the pain. One of the duties performed by certain Roman slaves was to remember whom their drunken masters spoke to at a banquet, what it was about, and how to contact him again. The slave who had this job was called a nomenclature. Epictetus's intelligence so impressed his master that he was eventually set free.

Once freed, he established an influential school of Stoic philosophy. One of his maxims was "no man is free unless he is the master of himself," which is something I've taken to heart in my long-enduring state of tentative health. I was already drawn to Epictetus because his chronic pain made me feel a connection with him across the millennia. I set out to master myself, specifically pain and the way I handle it. I believe that most of us live in dread of bodily suffering. We make every effort to avoid it, but we can't. At the same time, we ignore the suffering of the soul. Stoic philosophy became a way for me to transcend the suffering of my body, while attending to the needs of my soul.

Among the Stoics inspired by Epictetus was Emperor Marcus Aurelius, whose writings became some my favorites. His book *Meditations* is lively, simple, and direct. The edition I prefer has on each page a concise paragraph of wisdom. The experience of reading it was familiar, like reading a Catholic devotional—something I learned to do as a child and still do today. The core idea of Stoic philosophy was one I was ready to welcome as a companion to my catastrophic illness. In the words of Marcus Aurelius, "Very little is needed to make a happy life, it is all within yourself, in your way of thinking." I still carry a copy of *Meditations* in my purse and read from it every day.*

---

* Don't confuse this Marcus Aurelius with Marcus Aurelius Antoninus Augustus, better known as the Emperor Elagabalus, who invented the prototype of the whoopee cushion. He sat his lower status guests on inflatable pillows, and as the evening wore on, slaves would slowly release the air. By

The ancient writings of these Stoic wise guys helped set me on a path that would take me through the rest of my life, as I progressed from acutely sick to chronically, permanently sick. Stoicism is a practical philosophy. It stresses discipline and duty. The Stoics inspired me to meet the everyday challenges of my life and showed me how to deal with inevitable losses, disappointments, and grief. I have setbacks in my health and in my life. I get unhappy and discouraged. But an important tenet of Stoicism is that you become what you think about the most. Or as Marcus Aurelius wrote, "Our life is what our thoughts make it." I find Stoicism a great resource that fills me with resilience and vigor.

I later found echoes of Stoic ideas in writers from Friedrich Nietzsche to Ralph Waldo Emerson to Maya Angelou, who wrote, "You may not control all the events that happen to you, but you can decide not to be reduced by them." Sounds familiar, right? Or, as my other revered Italian philosopher Frank Sinatra put it, "That's Life."

Viktor Frankl's *Man's Search for Meaning* was another book that resonated with me as I began my life as a chronic pain endurer. He was a psychotherapist and Holocaust survivor who wrote about the possibility of finding meaning in life even in a death camp. "Everything can be taken from a man but one thing: the last of human freedoms—to choose one's attitude in any given set of circumstances, to choose one's own way," he wrote. Frankl's thesis is direct: life can be terrible, but

---

the end of dinner, they were under the table. Elagabalus married a descend-ant of the real Marcus Aurelius, and this is his only connection to Stoicism, but I thought it was worth mentioning because in addition to reading phi-losophy, I also enjoy making needlepoint whoopee cushion covers.

you alone have the control to decide what you think about a situation. When you are suffering, and you can imagine your life and how you will live through your suffering, this is your search for meaning. To search for meaning is to have meaning.

When you live with a chronic illness, you have to rise above mentality of victimization and feeling sorry for yourself. Suffering has been a stronger influence on me than all other teaching. Pain is intensified from trying to control what is uncontrollable. Acceptance and resilience have made me stronger. Adversity is a path to self-discovery. I am still in physical pain, but I try to not to have an emotional reaction to it. I have been bent and broken into better shape.

It is up to us to do what we can to minimize our pain, whether it's with medication, meditation, or exercise. Our desire for an easy life was taken away with our diagnosis; now we need the strength to endure our complicated new lives. Seneca, another Stoic, wrote, "It is the rough road that leads to the heights of greatness." I'm not expecting you to imitate Epictetus or Viktor Frankl; I'm talking about the greatness you can achieve in your own life. Be the best version of yourself. You're writing your own story now, so give it a happy ending. A lot may have been taken from you. But as Frankl wrote, "We are never left with nothing, as long we retain the freedom to choose how we will respond."

Of course the irony is that I only ignited my passion for Stoicism through competitiveness with my friend Mary. Envy, as Marcus Aurelius wrote, comes from "ignorance of real good." If I hadn't reacted from envy of my friend Mary's knowledge of the classics when we were in the gardens of the Sylvester Manor, I might never have bothered to go back and review Marcus Aurelius's *Meditations* in the first place.

On the basis of my appreciation of Stoic philosophy, I've developed my own pantheon of heroes, people who embody the idea that what impedes us can inspire us. They used the obstacles in their path as a motivator for success.

The people I will now introduce you to are four bad-asses who found the upside in having their lives turned upside down. They will forever be carved in my personal, imaginary Mount Rushmore—or as I call it, Mount Duffmore.

MOUNT DUFFMORE

Peg Leg Bates

For my most recent birthday, my husband asked me what I would like as a gift. I asked for a photograph of "Peg Leg" Bates, the one-legged tap dancing legend. His name was Clayton Bates until he lost his leg in a cotton gin accident in 1921, when he was twelve years old. His uncle carved him a wooden prosthesis, and he acquired the nickname Peg Leg. Against everyone's expectations but his own, he taught himself to tap dance. Peg Leg created an entirely new form of tap dancing, and his athleticism and dynamic moves made him one of the most famous tap dancers in the world. He starred in several films and performed on the *Ed Sullivan Show* nearly sixty times. Dixie Roberts, an esteemed tap dancing legend, said of him, "Peg Leg Bates danced better with one leg than anyone else could with two."

After Bates retired from the stage, he performed for the disabled community, for veterans, and for the elderly. His message was, "Don't look at me in sympathy, I'm glad to be me. I'm Peg Leg Bates and I unite hip gymnastics with dance fantastic. I'm Peg Leg Bates, the one-legged dancing man."*

Demosthenes

In ancient Athens lived a lonely, awkward orphan boy with a lisp named Demosthenes (pronounced "duh-MOS-thuh-neez." Now try saying that in Greek with a lisp). His guardians had stolen his inheritance and refused to educate him. He was tormented, bullied with no one to help him, so he helped himself.

Demosthenes moved into a cave and shaved half of his head to motivate himself to stay hidden until he reached his goals: educating himself and overcoming his speech impediment. He studied the great orators of his time, and to improve his speech, he stuffed his pie hole with pebbles and elocuted into the windy depths of the cave. He practiced reciting speeches in just a few breaths to improve the capacity of his tea-bag sized lungs.

Demosthenes eventually emerged from his underground lair, like Jesus and Punxsutawney Phil the Groundhog, and he announced that a change had occurred. He didn't seek revenge; he sought justice. He challenged his guardians in court and won back his fortune. He used his voice to right wrongs, and went on to become one of the most influential and legendary lawyers in Ancient Greece.

Florence Nightingale

Florence Nightingale was born in 1820 to an affluent British family, and could have lived a life of leisure. But by the time

---

* If you have never seen Peg Leg Bates dance, I encourage you to mark your place in this book and go to YouTube and watch old clips of Peg Leg.

she was sixteen she believed her calling was to become a nurse and care for people in need, at a time when nursing was largely a job for former (or current) prostitutes.*

In the early 1850s, the Crimean War erupted between Britain and her allies and Russia. There were no female nurses at the front, but after the appalling neglect of injured soldiers became known to the British public, the Secretary at War asked Nightingale to organize a corps of women to tend to the sick and injured.

Nightingale instituted sanitary guidelines and improved the quality of life for her military patients. She served nourishing meals, issued clean linens, and created a field library and classrooms for the soldiers. Her patients called her the Angel of Crimea and the Lady with the Lamp. Innovations put in place by Nightingale reduced the death rate by two-thirds.

While serving at the front, Nightingale contracted brucellosis, aka Crimean Fever, and by the time she was thirty-eight years old she was bedridden. She was homebound for the next fifty-four years. She could have whined and complained and accumulated bedsores and no one would have pointed a finger, as she had already devoted so much of her life to comforting the sick. But instead of giving in to her circumstances, she circumvented them. She dedicated her life to improving health care and alleviating the suffering of others, even as she endured a painful, chronic illness. She worked from her bed and wrote thousands of articles about health care reform, and today she is revered as the mother of modern nursing.

---

* During the Civil War, General "Fighting" Joe Hooker increased his troops' morale by allowing prostitutes to have access to his soldiers. These ladies of the night became known as "Hooker's girls."

Theodore Roosevelt*

Theodore Roosevelt, our twenty-sixth president, was the youngest man ever to become president (at the tender age of forty-two) and is remembered as a vigorous outdoorsman. Yet he was a weak, sickly child. His asthma was so severe that he could not attend school. His parents tried various remedies of the time, such as having little baby Theodore drink strong black coffee and smoke cigars. His father also took him on wild nighttime carriage rides through New York City; the idea was that screaming in terror would engage and strengthen his lungs.

Finally, his father said, "Theodore, you have the mind but you have not the body, and without the help of the body the mind cannot go as far as it should. I am giving you the tools, but it is up to you to make your body." Young Theodore responded, "I will make my body."

His father built a gym in their home, and Theodore devised a strenuous health regime involving medicine balls, the juggling of Indian clubs, and bare-knuckle boxing. His asthma improved, and he was able to attend Harvard, where he boxed and rowed on the crew team. He vowed to live each day with vigor and dedication to improving himself.

As a child during the Civil War, Theodore witnessed first-hand the draft riots in New York. The wanton violence made such an impression on him that he dedicated his life to protecting the weak and the powerless, having known what it felt like to be weak and powerless.

When his wife and mother died on the same day in the same house, Theodore didn't retreat into his depression. He

---

* NB, Theodore Roosevelt is on the actual Mount Rushmore as well as my Mount Duffmore.

moved on and went out to explore the Dakota Territory. His experiences in the wilderness moved him to later found the National Park System.

He served two terms as president and dodged an assassin's bullet while campaigning for a third. He was giving a speech and was shot in the chest, but the printed version of the speech was tucked into the breast pocket of his coat. The folded wad of paper slowed the bullet and saved his life— and he went on to speak for ninety minutes, as blood soaked his shirt.

Theodore Roosevelt was born a physically weak, chronically ill child, yet he taught himself to live what he called, in one of his best-known books, *A Strenuous Life*. I admire his fortitude and determination, although I have chosen not to smoke cigars or exercise with Indian clubs, nor have I earned the nickname "Locomotive in Human Pants."

I do share with Theodore Roosevelt (and with everyone on my personal Mount Duffmore) a love of books. When he was a child, Roosevelt taught himself to speed read, and educated himself by reading since he was too sickly to attend school. Cicero said that "a room without books is like a body without a soul"; Theodore had plenty of books, and plenty of soul. When he was president, he read a book every day before breakfast. In the evening, when he was done with official business, it was his habit to read two or three more books, in additions to magazines and newspapers. In a letter to a friend, Roosevelt mentioned over one hundred books he'd read in the year prior. The authors included Herodotus, Aristotle, Shakespeare, Milton, Dante, Moliere, Oliver Wendell Holmes, Sir Walter Scott, James Fenimore Cooper, Twain, Dickens, Thackeray, Keats, Browning, Poe, Tennyson, and Longfellow.

In addition to devouring tens of thousands of books in his lifetime, he wrote more than two thousand published works. I have tried to follow Theodore Roosevelt's example and am a constant reader. I don't know if I'll publish anything like two thousand pieces in my life, but Theodore Roosevelt is a source of inspiration.

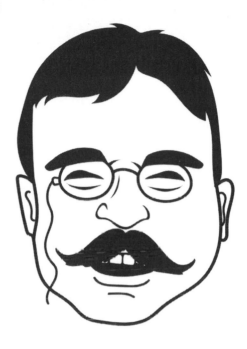

TEDDY ROOSEVELT'S SPEED READING TIPS

1. Review the table of contents and section headings.

2. Train your eyes to use peripheral vision.

3. Scan and skim, jumping over articles such as "a," "an," and "the."

4. Use your finger to guide your eyes along the page to avoid backtracking.

A STYLE FOR YOUR ILLNESS

MY HEALTH MAY BE going to hell, but I want to look good for the trip. The clothes we wear, the accessories we don, and the way we groom our hair and bodies—these sartorial cues send a message to the world about how we perceive ourselves and how we want the world to perceive us. There is power in how we dress. Epictetus said, "know first, who you are, and adorn yourself accordingly." I know who I am. I just don't know what level of pain I'll be in when I get dressed for the day.

When you're chronically ill, it's somehow possible to look scrawny and bloated at the same time. We want to dress as comfortably as we can, given our high level of physical discomfort. Some days we feel too distracted or too weak to care what clothes (if any) we put on. Sweatpants, baggy shirts, and flip-flops are just as much the uniform of a chronically ill person as a hospital gown. I'm not going to judge—go ahead, wallow. If you want to dress down all the time, I'm not the boss of you.

But your wardrobe is your personal archive—your sense of who you are. Anatole Broyard wrote in his book *Intoxicated by my Illness* that "every seriously ill person needs to develop a style for his illness . . . only by insisting on your style can you keep from falling out of love with yourself as the illness attempts to diminish and disfigure you." I think he's right. As your illness weakens your body, you can rely on your style to help transcend the insecurities and frailties that come with living with a chronic condition.

I'm not demanding that you squeeze yourself into three pairs of Spanx and wear a rhinestone-encrusted ball gown. But making an effort to look your best on the days when you feel the worst is well worth it. Broyard suggested that seriously ill people "buy a whole new wardrobe, mostly elegant, casual clothes." Well, maybe he could afford to. The rest of us have soaring medical bills to pay, and I for one won't be wearing couture and cashmere socks. But I do agree that it is important to stay in love with yourself when you feel like hell. Some may call that vanity. I call it the will to live.

Every outfit is a wish, a triumph of hope over experience. I want to stress that when I say "style" I don't mean you have to dress like you have Anna Wintour's clothing budget. I'm the last person in the world to go to for fashion advice. I was on *People* magazine's Worst Dressed List. I am in the coveted "Head to Toe Horror" category. I've tried to live up to the honor ever since.

When sarcoidosis first hit me, I developed granulomas in my brain and spinal column. Your skull is a contained space, and as the granulomas grew, they squeezed and then crushed the nerves in my spinal cord.

The granulomas shrank via chemo, but the nerve damage was permanent. As a result, I have chronic, unrelenting pain on the right side of my head and neck, radiating from the bottom of my ear, along my neck, to my shoulder and collarbone.

I can't bear to feel any pressure on my neck, so my hairstyle is always short. No beachy waves for me!

In my twenties, I got my hair cut at Nick's Barber Shop, by a one-eyed barber named One-Eyed Louie. His lack of stereoscopic vision gave me a slightly asymmetrical boyish haircut I favored. Louie had been cutting my hair for a few years when he suggested, "You'd be a good-looking fella if you got all of that hair out of your face." I informed him that I was a woman, and he told me to stick a sock in it. But there is a huge difference between a youthful, tomboy, gamine look and being addressed as "sir" in middle age. I lost most of my hair from chemo drugs, but now it's grown back into a style my brother calls "the Betty Rubble."

I can't wear necklaces, or any blouse or jacket with a collar that presses on my neck and shoulder. Soft, silky, floaty type blouses that slide off my right shoulder are the only type of top I can tolerate. So if I look like a cocktail waitress at a Pedro O'Toole's Cinco de Mayo Cantina happy hour—"Bailey's shots just one dollar! Fiesta like there's no mañana!"—now you know. My sister Kate disagrees; she tells me I look like a background performer from the '80s dance movie *Flashdance*, only way too old and a bit too fond of pie. I'm not here to argue. This is the style that suits my illness, and I have embraced it.

I'm a big believer in the maxim that it's a mistake to do nothing just because you can only do a little. This applies to the way you adorn your body. I will wear a dress instead of a sweatpants and a baggy sweater: it's only one garment to pull over your head, and you can find ones that are as comfortable as a nightgown. Slip on a pair of comfortable stylish shoes instead of sneakers the size of Easter hams. If sandals are your thing, try a pair that hides your corn chip toenails. High heels are now history, relics of my former life.

The neuropathy in my feet feels like I've got clunky mobile phones buckled to my feet, and they are constantly set on vibrate. My big toes feel like they're trapped in barbed wire tourniquets. Even when I'm barefoot, the duality of pain and buzzy numbness affects my gait. I may walk like a marionette with a tyrant yanking on the strings, but in my head I'm strutting with style.

I follow the rule of distraction. I pin a big gold monkey brooch with googly eyes on my jacket to draw judging stares away from my steroid-induced hunchback. My ultimate go-to accessory is a colorful, lightweight scarf. I can wrap it around my shoulders when I'm chilly; I can use it as a sling when my left ulnar nerve flares with pain. I tie it on my head when I don't have time or energy to do my hair. I loop it through my jeans as a belt if I've lost weight, or drape it to cover my chub and bingo wings when I've gained weight. I can wear it as a sarong or wrap up in it like a blanket. Can it even dress up a pair of baggy sweatpants? Yes! That would be a sartorial version of the mullet: stylish on top, scrappy on the bottom.

- -

HISTORY'S MOST DANGEROUS FASHION TRENDS

My hands are numb, and I've lost 80 percent of the use of my fingers on each hand. Zippers, buttons, hooks, shoelaces, and jewelry clasps are an exercise in frustration. I prefer to pop my head through the neck hole of a dress and wear shoes that slip on my feet. Long dresses and loafers can contribute to stumbles and falls, so I watch my step when I get dressed and so should you. Four people die annually from putting on pants, and drawstrings cause the most injuries of any clothing item. These fashion disasters put the killer clothes of years gone by in short pants. Summer Stevens' book *Fashionably Fatal* details what happens "when fashions are pushed to the extreme," a phenomenon she calls "vanity insanity." Among the crippling and deadly styles in her exhaustive treatment:

Corsets caused breathing difficulties and organ damage.

Crinolines, or stiffened petticoats that gave skirts extra volume, were prone to catching fire. Peak crinoline was reached in the mid-nineteenth century, which saw several high-profile and fatal crinoline skirt blazes. Oscar Wilde's two half sisters died of burns after standing too close to an open fire while wearing crinolines. According to the *New York Times*, in 1858 there was an average of three deaths by crinoline per week.

Men's starched collars were so lethal they were called "vatermorder," meaning "father killer" in German. The tight, stiff collars cut off blood supply in the carotid artery, causing death for men of all nationalities.

Hats. Mercury poisoning was an occupational hazard for milliners. The chemicals used to make the felt caused "Mad Hatter's Disease," whose symptoms were confusion, weakness, and trembling. Danbury, Connecticut was the center of American hat-making, and in the US the disease was known as the "Danbury Shakes."

Stiletto heels. The Chinese practice once practiced footbinding, a process in which the bones of women's feet were crushed together to produce a "more attractive" look. Today we condemn this practice as barbaric, but contemporary women are mutilating their feet for fashion as I write this. Pointy stiletto heels can be so restrictive that the only way to fit into them is by amputating healthy toes. One of my friends, a world-famous model, has punished her feet so thoroughly from a lifetime of wearing cruel shoes that she's had multiple surgeries on her toes. When she's barefoot at the beach, people stare at her gnarled, bony clodhoppers. She handles it with grace, and points to her boobs and reminds us, "The show's up here, folks!"

Muslin dresses. In the early nineteenth century muslin gowns were all the rage. To emphasize their figures (and show that they weren't wearing knickers), women would dampen their bodies so the muslin would cling to their curves. Damp muslin and cold temperatures led to respiratory illnesses like pneumonia, also called "muslin disease."

Chopines. The precursor to platform shoes, these extremely thick-soled and high-heeled shoes were popular in Europe from fifteenth to the seventeenth century. Chopines were up to three feet high. They were worn to help women step through muddy, dirty, sewage-strewn roads. Their height threatened mobility and one needed a cane or an escort to help walk in these stilt-like shoes.

- -

Women often fell off their shoes, resulting in injury or death. There is a strong link between clothing and mood. What we wear reflects and expresses what we are feeling. We tend to put on our favorite clothes when we are feeling good. It works in reverse, too. Putting on a special outfit will make you feel better when you're feeling low. Conversely, putting on schlubby old knock-around clothes can bring you down. It really is true that if you look good, you can feel better. My much better-dressed sister Kate told me that you should never go out of the house wearing an outfit that you wouldn't want an ex-boyfriend to see you wearing. Although I've been married for fifteen years and I'm dating much less, I take her words to heart.

You've probably heard that you should dress for the job you want, not for the job you have. By the same token, dress for the healthier self you aspire to, not the sick self you feel today. Even on the days when you feel horrible, I'll bet the rent that when you catch a glimpse of yourself in a mirror and see your favorite shirt in your reflection, you will feel better.

I find myself in the purgatory of a waiting room in the doctor's office or hospital at least once a week. I make an effort to dress up for these visits. I feel better wearing my favorite clothing, with my hair groomed, a bit of lipstick on, and maybe my toenails painted gold. I dress up because I like it and it makes me feel good, but I'm also trying to trick the doctor into saying that I look good. He's the expert, so maybe if he thinks I look okay, my health may be getting better. I'm fully aware that this is just a ridiculous mental game I'm playing with myself, but it uplifts my mood. I'm not above a bit of psychological trickery to keep my spirits up.

A doctor's waiting room is full of desperately sick people in catastrophic pain. When I was truly at my worst and visiting specialist after specialist in search of a diagnosis, I would check out the other patients. I was looking for someone who looked hopeful. Someone who looked like they had a life outside of the hospital. Part of the reason I dress up for my doctor visits now is if some newly diagnosed person is searching for a ray of light in the waiting room, perhaps they can get a wee bit of inspiration from me. "Hey, that person looks like she's holding it together. Maybe there is hope for today." I have no idea if I'm helping. But I'm giving it a shot. Waxing my mustache isn't going to change the world, but it will make me feel better about myself. If I reflect a bit of positivity in a scary waiting room, then I'm cool with having hot wax ripped off my upper lip. As Elizabeth Taylor said, "Pour yourself a drink, put on some lipstick, and pull yourself together."

THE LIPSTICK EFFECT

If you're a man impatiently waiting for a woman to finish her makeup, you can fill the time by learning just how important lipstick really is. As far back as the Roman Empire, wearing red rouge on your lips was a symbol of high social status. During the Great Depression lipstick sales increased as people comforted themselves with small luxuries. More recently, researchers at Harvard University have found that women wearing lipstick were perceived as more competent and reliable.

I don't take my illness too seriously. It is a serious illness, but my coping strategy is to find humor in the humiliations. When I broke my foot for the third time in a year, I spray painted my cast metallic gold, propped myself up with a gold glitter-speckled cane, and went to the Golden Globes Awards as the wingman for a pal who was nominated. I also wore a flask bracelet filled with bourbon, which is an essential accessory for the sick *and* the well.

Sir John Wheeler-Bennet wrote that "circumstances determine our lives, but we shape our lives by what we make of our circumstances." When sarcoidosis attacks another organ, I am challenged by yet another obstacle my unpredictable disease has placed between me and what I want to accomplish with my life. My doctor just told me that I need eye surgery—and surprise, this new problem has nothing to do with sarcoidosis. I was in disbelief and didn't know how to respond. I took a few steps towards acceptance by going on eBay and buying a vintage lorgnette—the kind of opera glasses used by Margaret Dumont, the straight woman in the Marx Brothers movies. They're on a stick you use to hold the lenses up to your eyes, rather than hooking over your ears. My new lorgnette has rhinestone-encrusted cat's-eye frames, and they make me feel a little better about the scary new problem with my vision.

I live around the corner from a party store that has a huge selection of pranks and practical jokes, so I bought a pair of glasses with spring-loaded eyeballs that pop out. This morning I hid behind the newspaper and complained about the pain behind my eyes. When my husband came into the dining room to kiss me goodbye, I poked my head out from behind the paper with two googly eyes. I think he appreciated it. Later today I'm going to start embroidering an eye patch with a winking eye, so after my surgery I can adjust to monovision my way.

When I lost most of my hair from taking a chemotherapy drug, I didn't go the tasteful route with artificial hair. My buddy

Jon and I went shopping at a Greenwich Village drag queen supply store. We bought a matching pair of enormous Afro wigs, and Jon wore his in solidarity with me. We decided to go to the movies after wig shopping. I may have overcompensated in the hair department, as the usher asked us to move back a few rows because other theatergoers could not see over our wigs. I never wore a conventional hair replacement. All my wig choices were novelties, like a waist-length Cher wig I bought to wear to my best friend's engagement party. This particular choice kept slipping off my head, so I kept it in place with tape and the chinstrap of a kid's cone-shaped paper party hat.

- -

WIG THIEVES

In eighteenth-century England, another thing to worry about besides cholera, smallpox, and rickets was getting your hair heisted by wig snatchers. Powdered wigs were prized among the royal court and upper class. The higher your towering wig, the higher your social standing. Wig thieving tactics included training monkeys to steal wigs off of highborn heads. Or small boys hiding in baskets would jump out, startling the wig-wearer, and the boys would toss the dislodged hairpiece to a trained dog.

- -

I could take up permanent residency in my couch fort, or I can accept my limitations and bull my way through. My style is to appreciate what I have and don't get too worked up over what I don't have. Marcus Aurelius wrote, "Put from you the belief that I have been wronged and with it will go the feeling.

Reject your sense of injury, and the injury itself disappears." I have rejected the image of myself as an injured person. Even when I'm racked by nerve pain and have one bad eye and one not so good eye, I think of myself not as an incomplete invalid, but as a complete Cyclops who is dealing with the impact of my illness the best way I know how.

MUSTACHES ON A STICK

Cut out your favorite mustache and tape it to a straw or tongue depressor. Voila! An instant disguise for doctor's rounds or visitors.

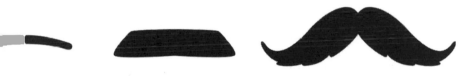

THE DUFF   PORNSTACHE   THE ROOSEVELT

WELCOME BACK, MR. KOTTER   WILFORD BRIMLEY

HAVE MERCY

WHEN MY SON WAS about to begin kindergarten, I decided to go back to school as well. I'd gotten a second shot at life, and that included the gift of being a mother. But I wanted to give back some of the love and care I'd received during my acute illness. I wanted to do something I was good at and that served others as well.

When Lefty entered school, I enrolled in a course to become a hospital chaplain. My goal was to provide palliative care and comfort to grievously ill people and their families. It was a kind of service I thought I'd be good at, having worked in nursing homes for years. I had the bonus experience of being the primary caretaker of extremely aged and extremely difficult relative. Plus, being chronically ill gave me a leg up on connecting with bed-bound patients. I was hoping that volunteer work would give me a bond with committed colleagues, as well as the satisfaction of doing something useful, beyond the limits of my daily occupation as a chronic invalid.

In our first day in chaplaincy school, our teacher, a Zen Buddhist priest, asked why we were interested in becoming chaplains. One of my fellow students was a very handsome gentleman in his seventies, pulled-together and professorial.

He said, "I'm drawn to chaplaincy, specifically Buddhist chaplaincy, because it's cool. I'm a single guy and it gives me something interesting to talk about. It makes me seem like a serious and caring man."

I secretly applauded and high-fived this guy for bringing up an important question: Is there such thing as true altruism? At what point do we decide to volunteer as proof to others that we are good people? When does volunteering just seem like a good PR move?

I was raised in a family where service was valued. My parents welcomed foster children into our home, and sponsored a family of refugees. Our parents encouraged all of us to believe that service is the rent we pay for life on earth. My dad always said if you do something kind for another person and anybody else finds out about it, it doesn't count. (I hope he was wrong, because now everyone reading this book knows about what my family did, and I'd like it to still count.) If there is a selfish element to my altruism, so be it—I'm still trying to do my best.

The chaplaincy school combined classroom teaching with field experience in a hospital. I spend a lot of time in hospitals, so I thought I'd be on comfortable ground. But during the first weeks as a student chaplain, one of my teachers pointed out that I was actually reluctant to knock on patients' doors.

I thought I was being discreet, but after I gave it some consideration, I realized the reason I was uncertain about knocking on a patient's door. When I'm an inpatient, the last thing I want is a stranger bothering me when I'm trying to rest in my hospital bed. Who needs a gasbag in your room flapping their gums when you're trying to get some shuteye?

"Not everyone has the same feelings you do, Duff," my teacher said. "And not everyone has a loving family and a lot of friends who come to visit. Many people are alone except for the hospital staff. They want to talk to people. They want to talk to you."

My teacher said he was going to watch me like a hawk to make sure that I did knock on doors. I doubted my decision to study to become a chaplain. I assumed I could just silently walk around the halls and pray for all these people who were suffering. Pray for strength, for them and for their families. Preferable from the privacy of a broom closet, or under a tarp in the part of the hospital that was under renovation. I really felt I did my best work from my hidey-hole. My vision of service didn't include actual contact with actual people.

When I have to check into the hospital, I often pack my collapsible kayak paddle. I'm frequently in the neurology ward, where the other patients have critical illnesses, including dementia. Some of the dementia patients are called "sundowners," which means that they get all fired up as the sun sets each night. And since I am usually tethered to an IV full of steroids, I keep my kayak paddle near my bed so I can reach over and slam the door to keep people out. It works just as well to slam the door on well-meaning but unwanted daytime visitors, too.

But my teacher was right. Not everyone is like me. Not everyone packs a kayak paddle when they go to the hospital. So I gathered up my courage and the charge nurse gave me a short list of patients to visit on the oncology ward. I gently tapped on a patient's door. I asked the fortyish man inside if he'd like a visitor. He invited me into the room, and I took a cautious step forward.

"Hello, I'm Karen Duffy, but most people call me Duff. I'm a student chaplain."

He shook his head. "I can't hear you, can you come closer?" It wasn't a private room, and the other occupant had the TV blaring, in addition to serenading us with an intestinal aria.

I click-clacked toward his bed in my knee high boots. I was so focused on projecting a positive, confident impression, I didn't notice this guy was attached to a plastic bag into which his urine was draining. Usually these bags of urine hang somewhat discreetly off the side of the bed. This one was so full, it was stretched to its limits and was lying on the floor. I accidentally stomped on the bag with my pointy boots, sending up a geyser of urine back up the tube that soaked the bed linen and my new friend.

"Did you do that?" I blurted in panic. I tried the old blame the victim trick—not very chaplainesque. It was then that I noticed the patient's brother, who had witnessed the whole thing from his seat on the windowsill.

The brother stared at me. He started cracking up and asked, "Are you the girl from *Dumb and Dumber*?"

"Yes, I was in the movie *Dumb and Dumber* . . . a long time ago," I admitted.

He asked, "Is this a prank? Did one of our friends arrange to have you punk us?"

I explained that chaplaincy students have a pretty small playbook when it comes to pulling practical jokes on hospital patients. I was new at this, I explained, and I was nervous.

I rang for the nurse, and both of us got cleaned up. I bowed my head partly in embarrassment and in part to hide my risorius of Santorini. This is a facial tendon that pulls my face into a natural smirk. It is often called "Santorini's laughing muscle." Not everyone has this. It's the opposite of what people now call "resting bitch face," in a person whose everyday expression seems sour and unhappy. My resting expression is a snarky smirk. The risorius has always been a problem for me at serious moments. I got reprimanded by the nuns in grade school for smiling, and sometimes I wasn't. I get it—I get tired of my leering mug too. This is the risk of the risorius. Oliver Wendell Holmes Sr., the polymath, writer, and humorist, found the risorius of Santorini particularly irksome in an acquaintance. He wrote that if he had one himself "I would have it cut out of my face." I'm with Holmes on this one, but so far I haven't found a doctor willing to do the deed.

I made a point of visiting this guy every week. Months later, I ran into his brother on the subway. He said that the story of me popping his brother's urine bag is now a family legend. Hospital chaplains are supposed to aid and comfort patients and their families as they near the end, and I guess I wound up doing that, just not in the way my teachers had tried to impart.

I was committed to the chaplaincy course for a year. I took additional workshops on the end of life and caregiving to the caretaker. I went to classes on the weekends and did my internship hours at the hospital. I wrote monthly papers and a final thesis. These rituals actually strengthened my commitment to the coursework. The reason volunteering feels so good is that without an obvious external reward, we create an internal reward system—in my case, I was giving myself brownie points for just trying to be of service. I believe in giving yourself for the greater good, and I know that altruism is not detached from personal gain. But my desire to become a chaplain began to seem selfish. I didn't have the correct skill set, or temperament, or even the right face for it.

Kurt Vonnegut once said, "We are what we pretend to be, so we must be careful about what we pretend to be." I decided to stop pretending to be a hospital chaplain, because I was pretending to be a bad one.

Looking back, I don't know why I chose to work in a hospital. Even though I've been in and out of them for the past fifteen years, I can't stand the sight of blood, or any other bodily fluid. I have a lightning-quick gag reflex, so the sight of a gigantic goiter, tumor, weeping sore, or other visible sign of illness makes my stomach turn. This is a drawback when you're supposed to minister to dying people, because death can be messy. The one thing I had going for me was that I have no sense of smell. I would bargain with the other chaplaincy students and offer to visit the olfactorily challenged patients. Unfortunately, there weren't many patients who both smelled bad and didn't have some type of visible bodily affliction.

My doctor had warned me that my immune system had been compromised by years of chemotherapy and that I should spend as little time as possible in hospitals, especially when I wasn't there for treatment myself. I was a little relieved to take his advice. I don't beat myself up for washing out of chaplaincy—I've found other ways to be of service. And when you've got a chronic illness that's always lying in wait to pummel you like a schoolyard bully, it's foolish to beat yourself up too.

The hospital closed right after my tenure as a student chaplain, and I felt like I was off the hook. But the classroom and clinical education was invaluable. I learned so much from the experience. I'm still very close to my teachers, and I used the lessons of compassion they imparted in every area of my life. Part of the training was to write a final thesis paper and give a presentation to the class. I had been inspired to take the chaplaincy course after reading Terence Ward's masterful book *The*

Guardian of Mercy, about the painter Caravaggio and his altarpiece entitled *The Seven Works of Mercy*. The painting depicts the works of corporal mercy, and I took those as my subject. They are:

- To feed the hungry;
- To give drink to the thirsty;
- To clothe the naked;
- To shelter the homeless;
- To visit the sick;
- To visit the imprisoned;
- To bury the dead.

Caravaggio painted this monumental work in Naples while on the run from the law, because he had stabbed the thug Ranuccio Tomassoni to death in an argument over a tennis game. I guess he'd misunderstood another element of mercy: burying the hatchet.

When it came time to present my thesis to the class, I was nervous. I wanted to do well, and I knew that this was the end of the line for chaplaincy for me. One of my teachers had a major sweet tooth, and he went crazy for chocolate. So I decided to bring in a cake. I was the last student to give a presentation, at the very end of the day. I mentally bargained that even if no one liked my presentation, maybe they'd be happy to get a piece of cake. And I'd be feeding the hungry, one of the acts of corporal mercy!

I ordered a chocolate cake with white buttercream frosting and asked the baker to write "The Seven Works of Mercy" on top in chocolate icing. When I picked up the cake, I opened the pastry box to find that the baker had mistakenly written "The Seven Deadly Sins" instead. Which served me right, not only for trying to bribe the class with cake, which is Greed, but I was also on the hook for Gluttony and Hubris too. That's three of the seven deadly sins. It was also karmic payback for my lifetime habit of torturing my friend Lynn with inappropriate birthday cakes. Every year I'd pretend that I forgot her birthday and that I had to buy whatever the baker had left over in the pastry case. Over the past twenty-five years she has blown out candles on cakes that have read "Mazel Tov Moishe!" or "Happy Get Out of Prison Day, Bedbug Eddie"—never, ever a simple "Happy Birthday."

I sucked as a chaplain because I was afraid I was a bother. I wanted to be of service, and it occurred to me I could make good on the Seven Works of Mercy through other, less in-your-face, yet still important acts. Here's how I do it.

Feed the Hungry: In Caravaggio's painting, feeding the hungry and visiting the imprisoned are shown with one image: a woman, Pero, breast-feeding her starving, imprisoned father, Cimon. Umm, okay . . . how about not breastfeeding your own jailbird pappy? How about sending a check to a food pantry instead? Most charities and NGOs can buy in bulk, and they prefer money to canned goods. If you don't like people, donate to a pet-food pantry.

Give Drink to the Thirsty: Donate and encourage your friends to give to an organization that provides clean water where it's desperately needed. Charitywater.org is just one of many worthy groups. Or buy a round for your friends!

Clothe the Naked: My friend Genevieve wanted to work with children, and she donated her time at a group home for kids in foster care. She went after work and read bedtime stories. When she asked the caseworker where the kids' pajamas were, she learned that many kids arrive in foster care with the clothes on their back, and if they're lucky, a Hefty bag with a few personal belongings. Many kids didn't have pajamas and slept in their clothes. Gen decided she could help. She created the Pajama Program and set a goal to collect and distribute one million pairs of pajamas. To date, she's given away *four* million pairs. On any given day there are over four hundred thousand kids in foster care in the US. You can support the program by running a pajama drive, and the program also collects books to read at bedtime. I've been involved in the program since she started it, and on Tuesdays I read to kids at the Pajama Program reading room. What started as a way to get kids clothing has become a way to promote literacy, too. You can get more info at pajamaprogram.org.

Shelter the Homeless: Foster kids who don't get adopted live in group homes, or with foster parents. At age eighteen (depending on the state) these kids are basically out on their own. Foster Care 2 Success supports young adults who've aged out of the foster system and are now going to college or technical school by connecting them with mentors via email, helping them to get an education that will keep them from ever being homeless again. FC2S also runs something called the "Red Scarf Project," which sends hand-knit scarves as part of a Valentine's Day care package, because former foster kids don't get gifts from home. I can't knit because I lack the dexterity, so I organized a scarf drive. You can always find a way to be useful.

Visit the Sick: Chemo Angels is a great organization that helps you become a pen pal with cancer patients undergoing the rigors of chemotherapy. Something you may not realize unless you've been through chemo is that there are long periods of time where you sit around with an IV drip in your arm. It's a great time to read supportive letters. Note that your buddy will not necessarily write back. The American Chronic Pain Association also has a pen pal program, and I correspond with three fellow patients.

Visit the Imprisoned: Hour Children helps incarcerated and formerly incarcerated women reunite with their kids and build healthy, independent, and secure lives. Sister Theresa, the dynamic director, welcomes the support of volunteers with the day care center, housing, employment training, and mentoring. Several of my esteemed fellow chaplaincy students have moved on to work with Hour Children.

Bury the Dead: FEMA, the Federal Emergency Management Agency, makes disaster assistance available to help with funeral costs if the death occurs during a major emergency. If you want to help aid survivors in the wake of a disaster, http://www.fema.gov/volunteer-donate-responsibly is the place to donate cash, donate goods, or even volunteer your time. When I worked at the 9/11 Family Assistance Center, I was surprised to meet morticians from all over the country. They'd volunteered to help through the National Funeral Directors Association.

These acts of kindness are just a start. There are countless ways to be useful. The Dalia Lama said, "The prime purpose of life is to help others. And if you can't help them, don't hurt them."

SOBER SUE

In the early 1900s, the Hammerstein Theater featured performing dogs, monkey acts, and a human billed as "Sober Sue," the girl who never laughed. The producers offered a one hundred dollar cash prize to the person who could make Sue crack a smile. At first, audience members went on stage and told their funniest jokes and pulled their craziest faces. Then, professional comedians took the challenge and performed their best material. The act was wildly popular and it was a lucrative move by the producer, as the audience was entertained by the best comedy of the day.

No one ever won the one hundred dollar prize by making Sue crack a smile. The reason was not her poorly developed sense of humor, but because her face was paralyzed. She had Mobius Syndrome, a condition caused by the development of abnormal cranial nerves, which results in a mask-like expression. (It's similar to Nicolas Cage Syndrome, which causes actors to wear the same facial expression no matter what emotion the part calls for.)

Sober Sue was paid twenty dollars a week, which was a decent wage at the time, especially for sitting in a chair and not laughing. And in our modern age, Sober Sue could have had a very good career as hospital chaplain.

Permission Slip

I _____ ,

give myself permission to:

_____

_____

_____

LOVE THE CHUB

WHEN I WAS A model, I was never rail-thin. I was regular size. When I look at myself in the mirror now, I'd say I'm the size of a morbidly obese person who went on one of those extreme weight-loss reality shows and got down to what a heavy person would consider thin, and a thin person would consider fat. Most of the weight I put on was against my will. It's not like I guzzled fudge sauce and stuffed my pie hole full of cake. I really had no choice. I needed to take prednisone, a powerful steroid, to shrink the lesion in my spinal cord. I slowed down and chubbed up. My hourglass shape has added a few extra minutes.

It seems like most people have the idea that they have to lose "those last ten pounds." What if those ten pounds store all your compassion, generosity, kindness, and humor? Why would you risk losing all of that? You could turn into a humorless bag of bones, so why chance it? Imagine all the great things you could accomplish if you erased that mental recording that drones on in your head that you have to knock off that last ten pounds. Is it worth it that what you lose in weight you could add back in being a sourpuss? Think of all the great things you could do with this extra head space. Beating yourself up is not good cardio.

Nobody ever went broke underestimating a woman's need for self-improvement. A group of my mom friends go to "Boot Camp" exercise classes. I asked them when they were shipping out. I've tried yoga, but I can't stand sweaty strangers, especially when they're farting in my direction. People use the simile "sweating like a pig," but pigs don't sweat—it's humans who are crop sprayers of perspiration. I think my gag reflex got the biggest workout. Also, a crackpot instructor told me that "yoga will melt away your lesions," so I downward dogged my way out of his class. Besides, I noticed that the more yoga pants I had, the chunkier I got.

Friends have raved about cleanses and juice fasting, but I think that food is an important part of a balanced diet. My little sister did a seven-day juice fast and all she lost was a week of her life. Is it possible to do a liquid cleanse with vodka? I mean, it is fermented potato juice.

- -

EATING DIRTY

The word diet comes from the classical Greek *diaita*, which means "way of living," and the etymology suggests the reason modern diets don't work. People undertake a diet in the short term to lose weight, not as a long-term way of life.

The big diet movement now is "eating clean." There's a name for this obsession with eating organic: orthorexia.

I've got a much better diet I call "eating dirty." I propose that "clean" is actually the problem. If you really want to cut out sweets, empty calories, pastry, and all the things that help you pack your saddlebags, dirty it up. Drop it on the floor. Still want to eat it? Drop it on the floor in a subway car.

I bet when your cronut is covered with short curlies you won't want it any more. Voila!

You're welcome, diet industry!

One of the side effects of prednisone is that it creates fat deposits where you didn't have any before. I gained the dreaded truncal fat and grew the charmingly named "buffalo hump" on my back. I got Cushing syndrome, also known as "moon face." For a few years it looked like I was in a perpetual snit with my cheeks puffed out. Even the shape of my eyes changed. In photographs before I got sick I had a more rounded, wide-eyed look. (I was doing print modeling and TV ads for Revlon at the time, so there's an extensive record of my former face in old commercials on YouTube.) After two years of mega-intravenous doses of prednisone, even my eyelids gained weight.

Everyone agrees that steroids are tough. If you Google "prednisone is the devil," you'll see millions of hits. The side effects are no trip to the beach. But they are necessary medicine. I'll take prednisone again anytime I need it, and I am on a low dose right now as I write this. Maybe there's a positive spin on the side effects—like, how about if we look at mood swings as exercise? Or bouncing off the walls in a 'roid rage— let's count that as a workout.

One of my favorite German compound words is *kummerspeck*, which translates as "grief bacon." It describes the weight gained from comfort eating. It was coined during World War I, when many German soldiers died in battle and their grieving widows turned to eating to soothe their emotional pain.

Do people in chronic pain comfort eat? I don't know. Does Dolly Parton sleep on her back? I packed on enough *kummerspeck* to make breakfast for an entire peewee hockey team. Was my tea-time snack of a cup of Earl Grey and a whole sleeve of ginger snaps a fair reward for getting through a difficult day? Sure it was. And after a painful EKG, MRI, or spinal tap, I did look forward to getting out of the clinic and into my favorite diner, the Bonbonniere on Hudson Street in Greenwich Village, one of the last of the real greasy spoons. My brother says that if you eat there too much, your stomach starts to hurt before you order. French toast and a side of burnt bacon was my regular order. The real bacon became the grief bacon.

A pharmaceutical company hired me to talk about wellness and women's healthcare. I was taking several of this company's drugs, so it seemed like a fair exchange. My responsibilities were to speak to doctors at medical and pharmaceutical conferences about the patient's perspective on chronic illness. Having an illness changes you, and the primary and side effects of certain drugs will affect the way you look. My hair thinned out and my face puffed up, and my job was to communicate to doctors and pharmaceutical representatives the impact of these changes on the patient.

I was stunned when the PR director of the drug company called my agent to complain that I didn't look like a model anymore. I didn't look like a model when I was a model. When I am photographed with Cindy Crawford, we didn't look like the same species. I didn't look the same as before because of *their company's drugs*, and they had hired me to talk about the physical changes! My contract expired, and I parted ways with the company, to my great relief. I wish it was understood that sometimes the thing that solves one problem can create several new problems.

Around this time my agent, Peg Donegan, saw that a casting director was looking for actors, specifically a "Karen Duffy type." Peg sent me out to read for it. I didn't get the job. I guess I wasn't myself that day. But I'm in good company—I read that Charlie Chaplin once entered a Charlie Chaplin lookalike contest and came in third.

I realized the full extent of my physical transformation when I went to pick up a pair of brogues I had gotten repaired. My neighborhood cobbler shop is the size of a breadbox, and the shoemaker works in the back. He has a security camera pointing at the front door so he can see who's coming in, with a black and white TV screen at the counter, so any would-be robber knows that he's being recorded. I was waiting for the cobbler to find my shoes, and I looked up at his security screen. Another customer had come in behind me and was also waiting for service. He was a chubby middle-aged Asian man. I took inventory of this stranger, and the snarky fashion critic in me noticed that the floral patterned shirt he was wearing wasn't doing him any favors. I shuddered at his asymmetrical hairstyle, which was really dated. Even the lead singer of A Flock of Seagulls would have agreed it was a bad look. He had some kind of eyeglasses pushed up on his head, so maybe they were corrective lenses and he didn't see his reflection before he left the house. As I mentally ripped apart this stranger in the security camera, I raised my hand to push my hair out of my face. The portly Asian man did the same . . . and I realized I'd spent a good two minutes making fun of myself! I knew my body had been changing, but it was happening gradually, a day at a time, so it hadn't really hit me until then. My husband gets a kick out of making me re-enact this story at dinner parties.

Some of the changes wreaked by prednisone have receded, but I still have a bit more weight than before. I love to paddle kayak and flaneur; I just don't have the ability to spend hours exercising. I decided I should just make friends with my fat. We've spent fifteen years together, and so far it's been a rewarding relationship.

I have a friend—well, now I've downgraded her to an acquaintance—who always comments on my weight. At my birthday party I was also celebrating being released from a walking boot cast I had worn on and off for three years on alternating feet. Her birthday greeting was that I walk as slow as a turtle, and can't possibly keep up with my goal of ten thousand steps a day. I guess she was in a particularly helpful mood, because she also shared her weight loss and exercise plan with me. Honestly, there's nothing worse than a skinny person violating the sanctuary of your home by demonstrating squats. I took her advice and decided that I would do a reducing plan, too: I was going to reduce the time I spent with her.

I believe that my former friend's attitude is more about her than it is about me. She's actually disappointed with her life. She's endlessly striving for perfection, and since there's no perfect body or perfect life, she'll always be disappointed. She focuses on what she thinks of as my imperfections because they take her mind off her fears about herself.

Living with a chronic illness teaches you acceptance and resilience. It teaches you that perfection is a folly. I have embraced the chaos of my illness, and I have gratitude for every imperfect day.

I have aged, and I've thickened with my reduced activity. But I'm accepting of my body. We've been through a lot together. I focus on what I can do, not what I can't do. Perfection has never been in my vocabulary of self-descriptors. Instead, I am going to love the chub.

- -

THE KAREN DUFFY ULTIMATE WORKOUT

Most overeating happens at night, so instead of dieting all day, eat sensibly during daylight hours and diet after dark. In my book, you don't have to join a gym, either. And since this IS my book, here's my workout plan, with no monthly fee.

Reading this book for an hour: 100 calories
Laughing at the funny stuff in this book: 130 calories
Listening to music while also reading: 70 calories
One hour texting friends about what a great book this is: 132 calories
Talking to your family for an hour at dinner about this book: 140 calories
Eating dinner: 70 calories
After-dinner sex, perhaps inspired by this book: 120 calories

That's a total of 762 calories, the equivalent of jogging for an hour and a half, so don't feel bad about having dessert, too.

- -

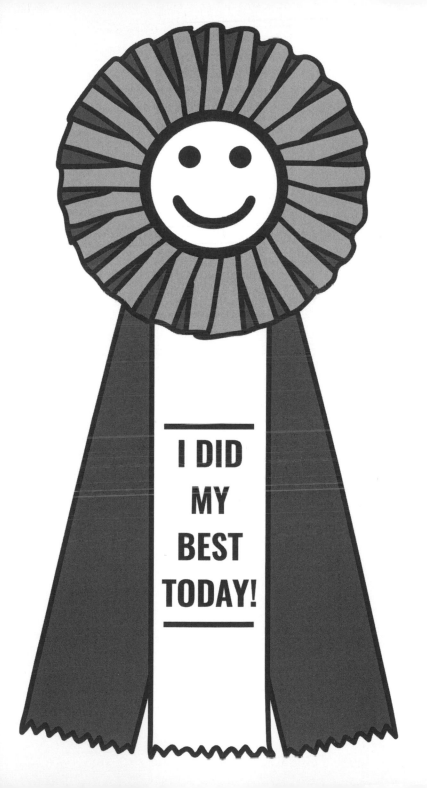

FIGHTING WORDS

I'M A FAIRLY UPBEAT person, but positive thinking is not a protective cure-all. Even the Dalai Lama can catch a fatal illness (I hope he doesn't, but some of his predecessors have). It's normal to be depressed, frightened, and angry when you're tormented by a major illness. There are moments when I'm so pummeled by pain, but it's not the relentlessness that makes me despair. It is hope that feels intolerable. But so far, I have survived every single bad day.

My nickname, Duff, is slang for getting a thrashing—if you get duffed up, you got beat up. Yet I'm a lover, not a fighter. I'm sick of sickness being described as a fight. Can we drop the combative language and war-like metaphors for disease?

Wars have winners and losers. When you talk about fighting off an infection or battling illness, you're implying that if someone gets healthy, they've won—and when they stay sick, they've lost. You often hear about a "losing battle with cancer." We say that people "succumb" to an illness, as if they gave in, and they should have "fought" harder. The not so subtle implication is that it's the fault of the patient that she could not "beat" her disease.

This belief has some ugly consequences. It suggests that the world is fundamentally a fair place, a meritocracy where goodness is rewarded and badness is punished. The belief in a grand plan fuels a bias in favor of the status quo—poverty, oppression, and inequality simply reflect the workings of a deep and meaningful pattern. The truth is that people don't always get what they deserve. Bad things happen to good people. Good things happen to bad people. And no amount of catchphrases will change that essential fact. Everyone is dying in increments. We're also dying in clichés.

Sometimes people will openly blame a patient for her illness. After the death of my friend Amy, I was walking down the street and ran into a woman who had been our mutual friend. I broke the news that our friend had died that morning. "I'm not surprised," this hag remarked. "She killed herself. She was so negative she gave herself cancer." I was shocked. "You can't give yourself cancer," I replied, "but you're gonna give yourself a broken nose if you keep talking like that."

Susan Sontag addressed this line of thinking decades ago in her book *Illness as Metaphor*. Sontag demonstrated that the language used to describe diseases such as cancer is based in the idea that the sickness is somehow the fault of the patient. When she was writing, quack psychotherapists claimed to cure the "cancer personality" that brought on the physical disease. Now, we have New Age snake oil salesmen claiming to do the same.

It seems to me the less you know about medical science, the more you will believe. It's easy to get misinformation via the Internet. As the meme goes, our invisible illnesses are more real than your imaginary medical degrees. There are plenty of healthy people telling us sick folk that all we need to do is fight harder. Instead of judging a sick person on their toughness or their attitude, how about supporting them instead?

Victim-blaming seems to be one of the last acceptable forms of public shaming. You don't say of someone who drowned in a surfing accident that "he lost his battle with the Atlantic Ocean." My friend who died in a skiing accident didn't lose his fight with the tree he skied into. If you go hiking and get eaten, it might be appropriate to say you've lost your battle with a cougar, but that's only happened three times in the last twenty years in the US.

When you have a serious illness, it's not a question of winning or losing. Some diseases are hard to cure. Some you can't cure. For some, the cure will be so difficult that you will never be the same as you were before. And some diseases won't kill you but will never leave you. The poet Nikki Giovanni had it right when she said about her own illness, "You don't fight cancer—you negotiate with it."

I coexist with my disease. The sarcoid-afflicted cells that cause me pain are a part of my body. My body is not my enemy. I want my days to be filled with love, resilience, and acceptance, and I accept that my life is not one of perfect health.

I am a Catholic. But when I hear "God has a plan for everything" or "God gives his biggest struggles to his toughest warriors," I want to serve up an un-Christian knuckle sandwich. I do not find my spiritual comfort in platitudes. I find my strength and comfort in family, friends, and service to others. I do not believe that my loving God is dragging us through a disease or a disaster in order to teach us a lesson about toughing it out.

The monarch of England, currently Queen Elizabeth II (long may she reign), is also the head of the Church of England.

Prayers for the Royal Family are a part of every Anglican service around the world. Someone once calculated that the British royals are the most prayed-for people in history. But they get sick and deal with mental and physical illnesses just like everyone else. Don't stop praying, but don't stop going to the doctor either.

Don't warm up that old chestnut, from Frederic Nietzsche via Kelly Clarkson, that "what doesn't kill you makes you stronger." It's true that you can grow in adversity. I have. I suspect everyone who has to face a major illness does. But if I had a nickel for every time someone told me "everything happens for a reason," I would be piloting my solid-gold submarine through New York Harbor.

In case it wasn't already clear to you, the platitudes and clichés of illness irritate me. I often hear sentiments like "you're so brave," or "it's a good thing I don't have your disease. I couldn't deal with what you go through." It's not like I signed up for this because I figured hey, I can handle it. I got sick because my immune system misfired and turned on me like a pimple-faced Judas. These are the breaks. When you get sick, you do what you have to do and go on as best you can, because the only other choice is a dirt nap. It has nothing to do with bravery.

I don't use the term "survivor" to describe my condition. I've been the chairperson of many Revlon Run-Walks for women's cancer research. I'm always inspired by the women who participate, whether they've had cancer themselves or are there to support a friend or family member. I've hosted the Survivor Ceremony at the finish line for fifteen years, and I know that in this community the word "survivor" can be an empowering one.

But calling myself a survivor is too final, as though I went through something and it's now finished. I'm surviving, but

I'm not a survivor. My illness it not over and never will be. It also feels like I'm fishing for a pat on the back, like I'm bragging. Look at me, I survived sarcoidosis! I'd rather encourage someone else than be congratulated.

Every day we are alive, we have survived. What do you want, the key to the city? What is it supposed to open? Actually, since a key to the city has no value and does nothing, that would be an appropriate reward. Congratulations, you survived another twenty-four hours. Your reward is that day and what you did with it. What matters is not *that* you live—it's *how* you live.

In the long run, we all have an expiration date. I'll never know when my number is coming up, so I've got to figure out a new way to describe myself. "Malingering endurer" suits me. Or "hanger-on." I've certainly gassed on plenty about my disease, so maybe I could describe myself as a "coattail rider of chronic illness." I'd rather undersell my situation.

When I die, I won't have lost a battle. I'll have won by the way I lived my life. I'm not combative. But when it comes to illness, the only thing I want to fight is the lousy way we talk about it.

WHY CANCER IS CALLED CANCER

My son was upset when he learned that his astrological sign was also the name of a disease. "Will I get cancer because my birthday is in Cancer?" he asked. I told him that Hippocrates, the father of medicine, had closely studied tumors in the human body (he called them "oncos," or swellings, hence our word "oncology"). Hippocrates observed that tumors with blood vessels radiating from them look like little crabs. He gave them the name "karkinos," Greek for crab, and that became the Latin and English word "cancer." The constellation Cancer, from which we get the zodiac sign, is also supposed to look like a crab. I don't quite see the resemblance myself, in either the stars or the tumors, but then, I don't see twins when I look at the constellation Gemini, either. I guess the ancient Greeks had more active imaginations due to the lack of distractions like season ten of *Finding Bigfoot*?

It's strange how our dread of the disease has become concentrated in that one word, cancer, that doesn't even really describe it. And I admire crabs, myself; they travel in their own house, and seem rather industrious and enterprising. I buy vintage enameled crab pins from eBay for friends with cancer as a reminder not to fear the word, not to give it power it shouldn't have. And as for my son, I've reassured him that astrology is just bunk anyway.

- -

- -

HOW BIG IS MY TUMOR?

My neurologist once described the large lesion in my brain as "non-caseinating." Casein is a protein in cheese, and caseinate lesions are soft and cheese-like. Instead, my lesion is granulated and more like an aged parmesan. But what is cheesy is the way we describe the size and shape of our tumors and lesions.

Wanda Sykes has joked that doctors use fruit metaphors because Americans don't understand the metric system, so a five-centimeter tumor has no meaning to us. Doctors describe your tumor as something non-threatening, like a peach or a ping pong ball.

It's pretty clear we need a new vocabulary to describe tumors, one that more easily and accurately conveys the appropriate level of worry. And I'm just the woman to devise it.

- There's a suspicious mass as big as a rat's hemorrhoid in your prostate. Let's keep an eye on that.
- You have a tumor the size of a viper's egg in your breast. I recommend a biopsy.
- Looks like a leech-sized lesion on your spleen. We'll need to remove it.
- I don't say this often, but the growth is the size of Hitler's dick. You'll need a course of radiation to shrink it, and then I'll cut it out.
- You've got a growth as big as an RPG on your colon. The best option is surgery, and then a round of chemo.
- The lump in your lung is about the size of a baboon's swollen ball sac. You should probably reach out to any estranged family members ASAP.

If the medical community insists on sizing tumors in comparison to something, how about carats? Everyone would know that a one-carat tumor isn't that big a threat, but a fifty-carat tumor is an invitation to get your affairs in order.

- -

EMOTIONAL BAGGAGE TAG

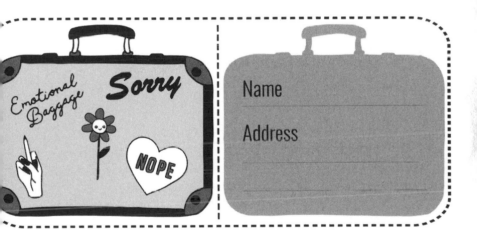

Name

Address

OUCH! PLATITUDE BINGO

WHEN I WORKED AT the Village Nursing Home, one of my favorite responsibilities, besides running the Frank Sinatra Appreciation Club, was calling the weekly bingo games. You haven't seen competition until you've seen a nursing home dining room filled to capacity with eighty geezers gunning for valuable prizes that included lottery tickets, lipsticks, and Tic-Tacs.

The level of competition was intense. No one suffered from memory loss on bingo night.

The bingo balls were in a wire spinner that looked like a hamster cage. I'd pull out a Ping-Pong ball, just like on the televised lottery drawings, and shout out the number. I made up silly rhymes and corny jokes to get the geezers all riled up. "B-9! Yes, I hope your tumor is *benign*, Mrs. Cella." If they only got out of their rooms a few times a week, I wanted to give them a big show.

I'd invite my actor pals to come and be my "Surprise Guest Bingo Callers." Comedian Chris Farley was always willing to help, and not just on bingo night. He once helped me take a van full of nursing home residents to a Knicks game and bought the incontinent old guys beer. Bless Chris. The residents of the nursing home didn't live their lives according to a book of affirmations, and Chris didn't treat them as cardboard cutouts, clichés of illness and old age.

In honor of my Monday afternoon bingo games, I have created Platitude Bingo. Platitudes are banal, trite remarks that are repeated to the level of pointlessness. But since most people are unfamiliar with illness, they fall back on these less than profound declarations. So why not make the best of it, and turn it into a game?

You can use pain pills or vitamin tablets as the markers. Every time a visitor utters a platitude or cliché that corresponds with one on your Bingo card, mark it. When you win—my website has a downloadable certificate suitable for framing.

OUCH!

You are in our thoughts.	Dr. Oz said...	You are brave.	How are you feeling?	It is what it is!
Why don't you try yoga?	Can I have some of your pills?	Eat organic.	Go with the flow.	Chin up!
When life gives you lemons.	Try acupuncture.	**Everything happens for a reason.**	God gives his toughest battles to his strongest warriors.	Look on the bright side.
If anyone can beat this it's you.	You don't look sick.	The only disability is a bad attitude.	We are praying for you.	You need to get out.
It could be worse.	It's just stress.	Tough it out.	Kale!	I don't trust western medicine.

TO WHOM IT MAY CONCERN

WHEN I WAS A kid, my cousin, a New York City police officer, was shot and killed on the job. I remember the phone ringing late at night, my mom's red eyes the next morning, and crumpled tissues shoved in the sleeve of her cardigan to help stem the flow of tears. My father was a police officer too, and we had many uncles and cousins on the force. I was scared. I remember feeling powerless.

I went to my room and wrote a letter to Richard Nixon, the President of the United States of America, the most powerful man on the planet, and asked him to catch the men who shot my cousin. I wanted to flip the switch myself on "Old Sparky," or press the plunger on "Old Injecty," whichever was in use at Sing Sing. (My position on capital punishment has changed since I was in elementary school.)

When you write a letter, it can change a life. I doubt the letter I wrote changed President Nixon's, but it changed mine. When the president wrote me back to tell me about the penal laws of New York State, I learned that if you write a thoughtful letter, you are not powerless. I changed because I realized I had power. I still have that letter; it's a valued possession I keep in the treasure box under my bed. My call for justice began a lifelong habit of writing at least one letter every day.

- -

A LETTER FROM THE PRESIDENT

The President of the United States gets one hundred thousand emails a week, and sixty-five thousand handwritten letters. You can request a special greeting for a birthday, wedding, anniversary, or retirement by writing to

The White House
1600 Pennsylvania Avenue NW
Washington, DC 20500*

- -

Written correspondence has waned in the past few decades. But I'm adamant that the art of letter writing should not shrivel with the advent of digital communication. Text messages are too short, too casual. Email is ephemeral and insubstantial. Does anyone save emails for years and reread them for their style, sentiment, and wit? I find much of social media to be immodest. If all I wanted to read were pithy brags and boasts, I could read my own journal.

A letter is a physical object. It stimulates all the senses— the feel of the paper, the rip of the envelope and the crinkle of unfolding paper, the shapes of signature, even the smell of

---

* The staff at the White House would really prefer you email them about this through the form at https://www.whitehouse.gov/contact, but the letter they send in return will be a real one.

it, especially if it's a perfumed note from a romantic correspondent. Even taste, when you lick the stamp, and the flap of
the envelope. (Israeli stationery has kosher glue for observant
letter-writers.)

A letter must be read, by definition, off-line—away from the
distractions of Facebook and your fantasy Lingerie League football team. And a letter, especially a hand-written one, implies the
time spent to write it—the care dedicated to a message just for
you. By the same token, writing and mailing a physical letter is a
simple investment you make for someone who really matters; you
don't use a stamp and an envelope to "like" the vacation pictures
of someone you knew slightly in college. A handwriting expert
once explained that if you look at brain scans of people while
they're writing, you can see that the brain lights up when writing
by hand, compared with a sort of dull twinkling when typing.
You're honoring the recipient of your letter with all the mental
attention and energy you've given to it.

Ernest Hemingway said he wrote letters because "it's such
a swell way to keep from working and yet feel you have done
something." Letter writing takes time, and illness has given
me an abundance of quiet time. I try to make the most of the
hours I am sitting in pain, curled up waiting for the pharmaceuticals to kick in. I may be physically slowed, but I take
inspiration from great innovators and thinkers who used their
down time to improve their minds. John F. Kennedy wrote
Profiles in Courage while recuperating from back surgery. Frida
Kahlo used her chronic pain as a muse and painted her self-
portraits while in traction. She painted her body casts and
turned her orthopedic aids into art.

I chose to write letters, which is something I can do even
at my most limited, and in letter writing I found a way to

transcend my homebound days. As Lord Byron said, "Composing a letter is a way to combine solitude with good company." I learned to accept the frustrations of the loss of certain physical capabilities, and feel connected and inspired instead.

Even when I'm feeling stronger, and I can get up and get cracking, I try to keep up my lifelong habit of at least one letter every day. I'm looking for someone to honor, someone to thank, some way to encourage. I send a lot of thank-you notes; I have a lot to be thankful for.

I believe my words are best conveyed by my left hand rather than by my mouth. I write to express encouragement, gratitude, or sympathy. A card or a note means so much more to a friend going through a bad time, or who has suffered a grievous loss. "Give sorrow words," wrote Shakespeare; "The grief that does not speak whispers the o'erfraught heart and bids it break." My dear friend and former landlord, author Richard Meryman, wrote that you must "wear out your grief just the way you'd wear out a suit of clothes." I hope my letters mean something to the people I wrote, but they are also very much letters to myself about my own sorrow, helping to wear it out.

Not every letter has to have a serious purpose. So I send kooky, cranky letters to the editor. Sometimes I write crackpot letters to friends, letters just to make myself laugh. I write my husband mash notes and hide them in his shoes so he knows how much I love and appreciate him.

Although my goal is one letter a day, on average I write much more. I order stationery by the ream. I buy stamps in rolls of one hundred. I enjoy funneling paper through the United States Postal Service, and I get a huge return on the investment.

I prefer to send several short notes rather than one endless eight-page effort. My advice is, just jot down thoughts and ideas as they come to you.* If you wait for divine inspiration to hit you over the head, you'll never post a letter. Visualize the person you are writing to, as if she were sitting across from you. If you have a doubt about whether to include something, don't. (This advice applies to most doubts, not just those about letter writing.) I never had a pen pal as a kid, unless you count President Nixon, but in middle age, I have many.

I read about guy named Joe Girard, supposedly the greatest car salesman in history, who sent his clients one note a month that simply said, "I Like You." If Joe were alive today, I'd write him back and tell him I liked his style. When a friend is in a sticky situation and I don't know what to say, I just write "I'm here if you need me." The mathematician Blaise Pascal once apologized for the length of a letter by concluding, "I have made this longer than usual because I have not had time to make it shorter."

At the beginning of this year, in the spirit of gratitude, I wrote a thank-you letter to every pharmaceutical company that makes a drug that keeps me going. To the company that makes a powerful time-release pain medication I take twice a day, I suggested that with all the terrible news about prescription pain medication addiction, perhaps they could use some good news. I have taken their pharmaceuticals responsibly and with gratitude. I love my life, and their drug makes getting out of bed possible. They wrote back asking to share my letter with their research department. I guess big pharmaceutical companies don't get much fan mail.

------

* Mother Teresa's advice is, "Kind words can be short and easy to speak, but their echoes are truly endless."

When you call, email, or text someone, there is a burden of reciprocation. When you send a letter, your recipient doesn't have the same responsibility to reply. This is helpful when your correspondent may not be physically or emotionally strong enough to write back. One of my best friends has amyotrophic lateral sclerosis, also known as Lou Gehrig's disease. She uses a computerized speaking board, and it takes her a long and tiring session to compose an email. Every week, I send her postcards and notes and bits of gossip, things we can share a laugh over, knowing that she can enjoy them without needing to respond. It's a small enough gesture, but it keeps us engaged with each other.

Remember that when you write a letter to someone else, you're also writing a letter to yourself. I don't expect a reply when I talk to myself, and I don't expect a response to my letters. It's the exercise of using my written voice that keeps me devoted to the practice. I understand that not everyone has a staff to answer the mail, like President Nixon. (Years later, President Nixon and his wife Pat moved next door to my parents' townhouse in New Jersey, and I'd wave to him when he pulled up the driveway. I don't think he realized it was me, his old pen pal.)

Then there are the letters I don't send. Oprah has popularized "gratitude journaling," writing down things you're grateful for in a diary. But after you write in it, that book just gets shoved in a drawer. I created a special journal to write letters to Lefty, my son. I want him to know how I feel about him, how I experienced his growing up and what I appreciate about him, and, of course, how grateful I am for him. I started writing to my son before he was even born, parenting for his future. I can talk to my brother and sisters if I want to go over our childhood, but

Lefty doesn't have any siblings, and I hope my book of letters will help make up for the collective memory deficit.

When Lefty was in kindergarten, his class made a calendar, and he was assigned to draw the picture for October. The pictures were to be unveiled on Parents' Night. When I arrived, Lefty led me to his picture. It was a portrait of me in the bathtub. A highly anatomically correct female figure featuring, just below the waist, a huge, out-of-control lady bush. I had been expecting a ghost or a skeleton for Halloween. Well, the picture was scary all right. It looked like a raccoon was sitting in my lap. October is a long month, which gave Lefty's classmates thirty-one days to discuss my grooming habits with their parents. This incident prompted one of my longest journal letters ever and the nickname "Crockett" from a few wiseass mom friends.

From these letters I never expect a response. I want Lefty to know what a great kid he was, and how thoughtful he was about having a sick mom. He never met me back in the golden age when I could turn my head and feel my feet. When stereoscopic vision was my view of the world. When my left hand was more than a crab's pincer. He knows me as I am. The letters I write to him are to remind him of his childhood, and in turn to remind me of how I mothered him. It's a two for one, and I always like a deal. This book of letters is a backup plan if Lefty doesn't get me as Mom as he grows into a young man. Long after my remains have been shot into the sky in a dazzling postmortem fireworks display, I hope my son is still reading my letters to him, so he can tell his children about his crackpot mom.

Find room in your life to write letters. Look for people to honor, to thank, or to encourage. You may feel powerless, but writing letters is empowering. According to the unscientific math of public relations, one written letter reflects the opinion of a thousand people, of the other 999 who were too lazy to pick up a pen. A handwritten letter carries the most weight. When an elected official receives hundreds of letters, it makes an impact and they take notice. Write a letter.

On the website that honors slain members of the New York Police Department is the Latin motto *fidelis ad mortem*, faithful unto death. I feel that in a small way, I keep faith with the memory of Patrolman Timothy Hurley with every letter I send.

I remain,
Your faithful correspondent,
Karen Duffy

ROALD DAHL

I've felt a connection to work of author Roald Dahl for many reasons. Dahl endured monumental injuries from a horrific plane crash while serving in World War II. He viewed his chronic pain as a "mental springboard" for his writing career. Dahl's imagination was never dimmed by the relentless physical suffering that was his constant companion for decades. His oeuvre is a testament to overcoming the obstacle of physical pain and giving happiness to the world through his books. He thought of himself as a "geriatric child," and I will admit to acting like a middle-aged teenager.

My son's favorite book is Dahl's classic *Fantastic Mr. Fox*. A few years ago our friend Wes Anderson was directing the animated film adaptation of the book. He wanted all the actors to live together and record the voices. My husband offered up our family farm in the Berkshires as the location. I was experiencing a fairly serious complication from sarcoidosis and was on bed rest for the month leading up to the week the gang was coming to record. I was weak and wobbly, but I remained inspired by Dahl, who didn't let his illness or pain stop him embracing the absurdity of life. Wes and many of the actors were old pals and I didn't want to let my affliction derail the fun. Dahl was a loyal friend, and I wanted to be one too.

George Clooney, Bill Murray, Wally Wolodarsky, Wes and his brother Eric Anderson, and the crew moved into our farm for a week. We ate together, drank together, and the guys bunked together in our guest rooms. Since I was still ailing, the guys pitched in and handled all the housework that as the hostess I'd normally want to do myself. George and Bill washed the dishes, made their beds, and washed the towels. It was heaven. I had a house full of handsome houseboys.

It was a week our family will always remember with great fondness, and I'm grateful we hosted the recording session. The week before everyone arrived I was in the basement and looked in at my late father-in-law's wine cellar. I thought, in our lifetime, we are never going to drink all that wine. After the recording session, we drank all that wine.

I even wangled a small role as Linda Otter. The puppet of my character that was used in the film is on my desk as I write this. It is a talisman that reminds me of Dahl's courage and fortitude.

Donald Sturroch's *Storyteller: The Authorized Biography of Roald Dahl* contains a gorgeous letter written by Dahl to his mentor, Charles E. Marsh. Marsh had contracted cerebral malaria and was catastrophically ill. Dahl wrote this masterful letter to lift his friend's spirits. It should be preserved under glass at the Smithsonian Museum as an example of the transcendent power of correspondence:

"I just want to tell you this: I am an expert on being very ill and having to lie in bed. You are not. Even after you get up and get well after this, you still will be only an amateur at the game compared with us pros. Like any other business, or any unusual occupation, it's a hell of a tough one to learn. But you know I'm convinced that it has its compensations—for someone like me it does anyway.

"I doubt I would have written a line, or would have had the ability to write a line, unless some minor tragedy had sort of twisted my mind out of the normal rut. You of course were already a philosopher before you became ill. But I predict that you will emerge a double philosopher, and a super philosopher after all this is over. I emerged a tiny-philosopher, a fractional philosopher from nothing, so it stands to reason that you will advance from straight philosopher to super philosopher.

"I mean this. I know that serious illness is a good thing for the mind. It is always worth it afterwards. There's something of the yogi about it, with all its self-disciplines and horrors. And it's one of the few experiences that you'd never had up to now. So take my view and be kind of thankful that it came. And if afterwards, it leaves you with an ache, or a pain, or a slight disability, as it does me, it doesn't matter a damn; at least not to anyone but yourself. And as you've taught me so well, that is the only unimportant person—oneself."

PEN PALS

It's hard to make friends when you're older, and life gets more complicated. We tend to cultivate the friends we met in school and early adulthood, and as we age we weed our social garden. Chronic pain can be isolating, and we thrive on connections. Great ways to meet people you don't have to explain yourself to includes the American Chronic Pain Association pen pal program, through the Foundation of Sarcoidosis Research, or at www.mycounterpain.com.

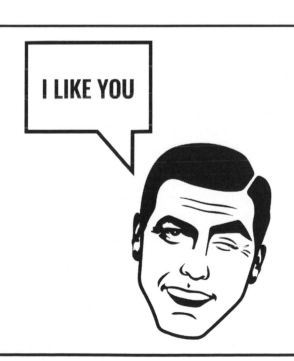

HOW NOT TO BE A JACKASS

THE BOOK OF ECCLESIASTES contains the proverb, "a faithful friend is the medicine of life." Good friends are good for your health. No doctor can write a prescription for friendship, love, and laughs. The power of friendship cannot be overestimated. It's up to us to be good friends to our friends. But some of your friends or even family members may be acting like jackasses, and making your tough row even harder to hoe.

People want the world to make sense. When a great person like you gets sick, it's not fair, it doesn't make any sense. You're a swell pal, why'd it happen to you? It can't be random, because that's too scary. If it's random it might happen to *them*. So these jackasses have to tell themselves a story, that you got sick because you ate non-organic gluten, or you work too hard, or you grew up in New Jersey. And you're staying sick because you're not doing what *they* bray. These stories soothe the fears your condition provokes in them. The healthy jackasses imagine themselves in the sick person's situation, and in their mind, they would be sick *so much better*.

REAL JACKASSES

I actually love jackasses. A jackass is the male of the ass species. A jenny is the female. The word "donkey" comes from the English word "dun"—referring to their brownish-gray color. The suffix *–ky* means small. So donkey means little dun animal. "Ass" is the ancient Roman word for my beloved animal. "Donkey" and "jackass" refers to the same animal. A mule is a male donkey—a jack—bred with a mare, a female horse.

This isn't just my theory. I often consult with a brilliant psychologist who studies the psychology of illness in women. She said that healthy people have difficulty conceiving what it's like to live with a chronic illness. They just can't face the truth that bad things do happen to good people, and sometimes it's random chance. If you get a chronic illness, then it could be possible that they could get sick too. And that manifests in jackassery (note: not a medical or clinical term).

Illness and pain are not character defects or signs of weakness. People living with autoimmune and other chronic illnesses are living proof that the human body is a fallible system. Life is imperfect. But victim-blaming has a long and venerable history. In ancient Greece, disabled people were blamed for calamities and cast out of their community. They were made into scapegoats—sacrifices who took the sins of the community on themselves, just as humans used to do with actual goats. My sarcoidosis isn't catching, but I did lose friends who just didn't want to be around it. They were too afraid of what

I'd become, and their fear made them angry, and their anger drove them from me. So I cast them out of my life. When your friends become a source of stress, it can be even more hurtful because you cared about them.

I went on a talk show to flog my first book, *Model Patient*. The host asked me about my childhood fear of leprosy. In my book, I wrote a single sentence about growing up Catholic, and how the illustrations of lepers in my children's bible scared the pants off me. It was just one line in a three-hundred-page book. I didn't even mention that when I saw the scene in *Papillon* where the leper's finger came off, it was all over for me. The host then announced on national TV that I'd given myself sarcoidosis because I was afraid of leprosy. I guess if I'd embraced the wholehearted desire to have leprosy I wouldn't have gotten sarcoidosis? And shouldn't I have gotten Hansen's disease, as leprosy is now rebranded? This talk show host had enough empathy to fill a teaspoon.

I got a letter recently from a woman suffering from a degenerative nerve disorder. She was often too physically exhausted to get up and around. In her letter, she asked for advice about dealing with her mother, because Mommy Dearest had her foot up her backside every day, saying she should be more active, "like that Karen Duffy." I wrote back to get her mother's phone number, and when I got it, I called to explain that her image of my life was way off. People only see me when I'm up and around, doing something in public. There are no cameras in my home. The only people who see me in my weak and compromised cavewoman state are my husband and son, and they don't browbeat me about being lazy when I'm unable to be active. I mean, they *mostly* don't.

Researchers have found that people with strong social circles have less risk of depression, and their risk of stroke and heart attack is decreased by 50 percent. A chronic illness can be socially isolating. The loneliness is difficult to own up to, and it's hard to explain. When you've got a chronic condition, you need the benefits of friendship more than ever. You know that; it's the jackasses who need to learn. Next time one imposes herself on you, you can read this chapter out loud. Better yet, have them do it.

It's easy *not* to be a jackass. Just reach out to someone. All you have to do is be present. Tell her, "I'm here if you need me." Proust wrote, "Let us be grateful to people who make us happy, they are the charming gardeners who make our souls blossom." Jackass or charming gardener—take your pick. When my pal was diagnosed with ALS, I was taking courses to be a hospital chaplain. After our kids went to school, I would go over to her house and study. I wanted to be there in case she needed me for anything, but also so she knew she was not alone. I knew she needed to mourn for the life she was losing, and I hoped that my unassuming presence would give her some comfort. I was not going to let her fall into a hole she couldn't get out of. We didn't talk very much, and that was fine for her and fine with me. I was close by and ready to help if she wanted it.

Chronic pain patients are thirty-eight times more likely to develop depression or other psychiatric issues. Because of the influence of therapy, aka "the talking cure," some people seem to feel that a constant stream of chatter is the answer for everything. Therapy is great, but I'm not your therapist, and you're not mine. A big part of being a good pal to a sick friend, instead of being a jackass, is knowing when to clam yourself.

There are some things you should never say to a person with chronic pain or chronic illness:

1. "Can I try your medicine?"

I'm in constant pain. I take very serious, strong pain medication that helps me live my life, but even with the help of morphine there are times when I just can't wear clothing or even get vertical. I need my medicine to survive, so no, you can't have any. It's no party to rely on these pills. Don't be an idiot and don't ask for them. We could die from misuse of these drugs.

2. "Everyone gets sick and tired. Don't be such a wuss."

When you're in pain, it feels even worse to let your loved ones down. It feels unbearable to not be believed. I am a patient advocate, and I write books and articles. I go around the country speaking about pain and healthcare issues. Yet some people I've known for decades can't understand that I have about 50 percent good days and 50 percent bad days. I get teased about gaining weight from prednisone—or just gaining weight. A woman I've been tight with since we were in out early twenties complained that I talk too much about chronic illness, and it will hurt my on-camera career. Um . . . what career?

3. "You look tired." "You don't look like yourself." "You've gained weight, Chubs."

Well, the chemo has really been taking it out of me. Thanks for noticing! And it's true the steroids aren't doing much for my figure. But I'd rather take my medicine than live up to your beauty standards.

4. "Keep me posted about your test results."

The last thing I want to do is discuss my personal medical information over and over again. Unless you are wearing a lab coat and I am paying you a bloody fortune for your guidance, I'll keep this information limited to my close circle of friends—and they don't need to ask. Sometimes it's a bummer to think about, never mind talking about it and explaining it.

5. "Let me know if there's something I can do."

I'm trying to manage my life and my illness—you want me to come up with your to-do list also? How about you use your noodle and figure it out for yourself? My sister Kate has a friend who was facing a long series of daily treatments for breast cancer. Her friend has a large family, so Kate and her circle of friends got together and bought a used refrigerator and put it in the woman's garage. On the door of the refrigerator was a list of what had been delivered and what was needed. When friends and neighbors drove by they would drop off milk, eggs, prepared meals, and household staples. This way the family had meals delivered to their door but they didn't have to deal with a constant stream of people knocking on the door, adding to their stress. If you want to help a friend in need, ask if there's something specific you can do—like walk the dog, mow the lawn, take out the recycling, or give her a whipped cream foot massage.

6. "Call me."

Why don't *you* call *me*? Then I can decide if I want to answer. I enjoy a chat as much as the next chronically ill gal, but when I'm down I don't answer my phone. I can't deal with the burden of speaking to anyone—it actually hurts to hold the phone up to my ear. If you call and I don't answer, send a card. I'll appreciate it.

7. "I'm not good at this. I'm so upset about your illness, I can't handle it."

Hey, jackass! It's not about you. I'm not asking you to donate a kidney. Having to deal with your dramatic overreaction is not helping. I have "friends" who act like my illness is the worst thing that's ever happened to *them*!

8. "You're sick because you work too hard."

Ugh, how the hell do you know? I could be a gold-bricking malingerer for all you know. I choose to fill up my life as best I can with things that make me happy: my friends, my family, working, and volunteering. It's not like I'm pounding rocks in a Chilean copper mine. I'm just living my life. These are the same jackasses who tell me when I'm bedridden, "You need to get up and around more!"

9. "Focus on you."

My spiritual and emotional fulfillment is based not on who I am or what I have, but what I can give. Many of my favorite philosophers have suggested that self-fulfillment is found through service. Who am I to argue with great philosophers? I'm a firm believer that life gives to the giver and takes from the taker.

10. "Don't take chemo, it's toxic—it's rat poison."

What *is* toxic is this type of comment from friends.

If you don't know what to say to someone who's been recently diagnosed with a serious illness, just acknowledge her situation. "I'm your friend. I know you are in pain. I don't know what to say, but I'm here for you."

Enduring a chronic illness takes a lot from you; it also takes a lot from your friends. Not everyone who was a friend is going to stick with you, or be the right friend for your new life. The five people you hang out with the most have the greatest impact on your life, so choose wisely.

I keep a pair of beloved four-legged jackasses at my farm, and I'm well acquainted with how to motivate them. I've spent a lot of time in this chapter wielding a stick, now it's time for the carrots—positive things you can say and do when someone's ill. Knowing how to behave will give you the power and confidence to be compassionate to a sick friend. Here are some quick tips on non-jackassery:

- Make eye contact. Don't act like you just encountered a leper you can't bear to gaze upon.
- Be supportive, even if you don't agree with how your friend is dealing with the situation.
- Be an active listener. Give your friend your full attention. Turn off your phone before you even walk in the door.
- Don't pretend it didn't happen.
- Don't talk too much about yourself.
- Think ahead: What do you think your friend could use? Can you bring pet food? Coffee? Some snacks for her to share with her other visitors? Stamps for letter-writing? If you do bring a little something, make it nice. I think people tend to skimp on gifts for sick people, maybe because they think they'll die soon so it's not worth it.

- Tell the truth. When you lie, the temperature of your nose increases and the redness is called the Pinocchio effect. By all means share the latest gossip—which can have positive physical benefits!

The isolation of a chronic illness can be as painful as the malady. Aristotle wrote, "A friend is a second self." Be second self to a friend in need.

PACE YOURSELF

When you have a chronic invisible illness, you have to practice pacing yourself. Our energy supply is not infinite. We have to prioritize our days and forecast how much energy we need to get through them.

Christine Miserandino, who has the autoimmune disease lupus, came up with what she calls the "spoon theory" to give healthy people an idea of what her life is like with a chronic illness. When you are a healthy-looking sick person, it can be confusing to the people we hang out with, our co-workers, and friends. She describes the units of energy needed to get through the day as being like a handful of spoons. Every task costs a spoon, and you have a limited number, so you have to pace yourself. Her "spoon theory" is widely circulated on social media, and a large part of the wellness community identify as "spoonies."

Here's how it works for me. Maybe I'm feeling rather run down on a Tuesday, and I've got enough energy to do ten things. Most healthy people can start their day by jumping in the shower, washing and then drying their hair, getting dressed, fixing some breakfast, putting on shoes, and then they're ready to head out the door. For me, taking a shower is a demanding, exhausting activity. In fact, I have to take baths because I can't tolerate water pounding on my neck. So a bath, that's one unit of energy down. When your arms are weak, using a hair drier is difficult. Two down. Trying to get dressed with hands hobbled by neuropathy—another unit. Breakfast for my family, even something simple like an egg sandwich or waffles—one more unit. Tying shoelaces would be another, but I'm already running low on energy so I'll wear slip-ons instead. Now it's 8:00 a.m. and I've got enough left in my tank to do six more things—and I still have to walk the dog, take my son to school, go to the market, write this book, check in on my volunteer projects, manage my small production company and my social life, and make dinner. As soon as I wake up, I have to decide how I really want to use my energy and make some compromises. (I usually skip the bath and hair drying, if you want to know.)

Instead of spoons, I prefer to measure the units of my daily life in something a bit less utilitarian. You could call it the "pizza theory." You get a pie a day, and only a certain amount of slices. Or the cake theory—it's how you cut it up. Or the wine bottle theory—you get six glasses from a bottle of vino and whether you sip it or guzzle it, it's up to you. Time and energy are precious. People with chronic illnesses have to ration them.

----

hello
my name is

I told you I was sick. Talk to me at your own risk.

EXCUSE DICE

When you live with a chronic illness, you will need to pace yourself. You will have to cancel plans and punk out on the people you love. It is uncomfortable to back out of social engagements. We feel guilty and selfish. But on the other side, as great as it is for you and your friends to get together, there are occasions where the nicest thing for them is to get a cancellation. They get a night off, too.

The hardest thing about canceling is coming up with an excuse, and it's boring (and slightly suspicious) to use "I don't feel well" or "my neck hurts" over and over. In the event that making up sniveling excuses doesn't come easy to you, I've provided the template for a six-sided die. When you run out of excuses you can roll the die and use one of mine.

Cut out the template and fold on the bold lines. Tape it together to create a cube, and you're ready to roll.

I just took a laxative and I'm not certain when it is going to blow. So it's better for both of us if we put a pin in tonight's plan.

BAD CLAM

I've fallen into a binge-watching hole and I can't get out.

Tell the truth, or roll the dice again.

My helper monkey got loose.

A hit man is looking for me. I need to lie low.

THE OPTIMISTIC CATASTROPHIST

Too much optimism can't be good for you. Leaping from one positive affirmation to another jolly platitude can make you insufferable to be around. How many stirring tales of grit and determination can you read before you make yourself sick (or even sicker)? I take my optimism with a healthy dose of catastrophism.

Living with uncertainty is a skill. My 103-year-old grandmother-in-law was bitter and outraged that her mild, age-related arthritis could not be cured. She could not accept that her body was aging and she was over a century old. Aren't we all on the greased chute to the grave? I accept that for me, it is pretty much downhill from here. I'm not perturbed; I am prepared.

I am an optimistic catastrophist. I believe things are going to be great, until they aren't—and at that point things will go off the rails in a spectacular disaster. Healthy people have what's called "normalcy bias"—because serious health issues haven't happened to them, they imagine that they never will. Living with an unpredictable illness gives you a heightened awareness of looming catastrophes, so it's up to me to make the best of things before they go sideways. Embrace the chaos of the unpredictability of life and live it up while you can. Pie-eating contest followed by upside-down margaritas? Don't mind if I do! Naked kayak races in a phosphorescent tide? Count me in!

We assume that the greater the trauma, the greater the suffering and enduring distress. This is not always the case. In a study titled "The Peculiar Longevity of Things Not So Bad" by Dr. Dan Gilbert, he and his team of researchers found that when spectacularly bad things happen, our brains compensate to aid our emotional recovery. Sometimes minor setbacks can throw you into despair and can induce longer-term distress than major disasters. Sometimes we can recover more easily from a big fight with our sister than from getting stink-eye from a complete stranger. This anomaly is called the region beta paradox.

Dr. Gilbert also found that participants recovered faster from an insult directed at them personally. When an insult was directed at someone else, the participants took longer to recover. Dr. Gilbert believes that when we are personally emotionally pained, we can protect ourselves with obfuscation and excuses. Our self-preservation instincts kick in. When we witness other people suffering, our empathy ignites. In other words, seeing you in pain causes me pain. I suppose this is what my mom meant when she threatened me with the "Spanking Spoon" and said, "This hurts me more than it hurts you." I believe this can explain the resilience of some people who've been struck with health issues—paradoxically, it's easier for the patient to get over complications and downturns than it is for her friends and family.

Chronic pain, like other types of suffering and discontent, can tempt you to withdraw and turn inward. But solely focusing on your own obstacles and problems does not help you or anyone else. My dad likes to say, "A big problem in life is that people expect there to be no problems in life." I expect complications and anticipate negative side effects. As Aristotle wrote, "It is likely that unlikely things should happen."

I am grateful for my life, and I want to give back. I want to learn skills that will allow me to be useful, even if it's only in a small way. Citizenship confers obligations as well as rights. My desire to be useful gets stronger as my body gets weaker. These setbacks do not deter me from my goal.

There are many ways to step up and help others in need. We all can't run into a burning building when everybody else is running out. We all can't do monumental, heroic deeds. Mother Theresa said, "We all can't do great things, but we can all do small things with great love." I find inspiration in this quote every day. We all have a choice, to be useful or useless. I try to be useful.

The word compassion means "suffering together." Viktor Frankl suffered and lost his entire family in the Nazi death camps. Yet he found meaning through caring for his fellow inmates. I believe that to the degree you are helpful to others, you will find a way to contentment. No one has a perfect life. Everyone has problems and faces challenges. It's up to us to find meaning in them.

The word "disaster" is derived from the ancient Greek words "dus," meaning bad, and "aster," meaning star—so, "bad star." The word comes from the astrological sense that a catastrophe is caused by the position of the planets. Doesn't it seem like the ancient Greeks were always blaming something else when things went wrong?

Disasters show us what we are made of, and they also show us what other people are made of as well. In the book *Survival*

Psychology by John Leach, he described three types of reactions to catastrophe. In an extreme emergency, 10 percent of people will completely lose it and make a bad situation worse. 80 percent will go into a kind of stunned shock and behave in a robotic manner. They'll go along with a crowd, or respond to instructions, but won't take initiative (also known as "the bystander effect"). The final 10 percent of the population with handle a crisis with a rational mindset. They can assess the situation, develop priorities, make a plan, and take action. The ability to keep your cool and not get overwhelmed is called "splitting." I was determined to teach myself to be like the people in this aspirational 10 percent.

When I learned that New York's Office of Emergency Management was forming volunteer units called Community Emergency Response Teams (CERTs), I signed up right away. I already felt attuned to things that might go wrong because of the unpredictability of sarcoidosis. I have to be prepared for pain flares and rare side effects of my illness. I always carry extra pain medication. I keep in my wallet a laminated card with information about my condition and my drug protocol and who to contact if I keel over. It is said that in New York City you are never more than six feet from a rat. I am never more than six feet from a rattling bottle full of medication.

I was taught as a child that if you fail to prepare, you prepare to fail. As an adult, I always identify the emergency exits in airplanes, theaters, and subways, and make my son count the doors to the stairwell whenever we check into a hotel. I was prepared to help myself and my family, but I wanted to be useful to my beloved city and the proud sons and daughters of the Empire State. I wanted to be like my Office of Emergency

Management teachers—a good person to have around when things don't look so good.

The OEM teachers trained our team in CPR, triage assessment, first aid, traffic control, and other skills so we could support the work of the first responders. We learned how to help the public in case of any disaster that might befall New York. I learned to keep a small first aid kit in my purse—just a ziplock bag with hand sanitizer, Band-Aids, alcohol wipes, latex gloves, eye drops, aspirin, a small flashlight, and mints. A flashlight is good if you're stuck navigating a dark building or subway car. Plus, the smoking hot NYC fireman who taught the course said that having a source of light is comforting, and I was happy to follow his advice. I learned that mints are great to pass around as well, especially if you're trapped in a dark elevator with someone who had a chili dog with onions for lunch. A good rule of thumb is never turn down a breath mint—it's being offered for a reason.

My excellent Office of Emergency Management training has taught me I can be useful instead of useless. Our Manhattan Community Board 2 CERT Team has a lot to offer. A few of us live with chronic illnesses, and some of our team members are senior citizens. One or two have mobility issues, and one even uses portable oxygen bottles. But one of the great things I learned from being a part of a team is that there is a job for every kind of person. After all, I've got my own limits, but I think of myself as an AMP—able-minded person.

My grandfather was a part of the New York City Civil Defense in Greenwich Village during World War II. Seventy years later, I was proud to follow in his footsteps, just blocks away from his Perry Street apartment. I serve the same neighborhood; I even have an official helmet and vest to wear in emergencies, just like my Grandfather Duffy.

There's a psychological process called the "Baader-Meinhof phenomenon," also known as a "Frequency Illusion." When you learn something new and unusual, you start spotting examples of it all around you. Your brain is primed to notice this new bit of information, so you have the impression that the new thing is suddenly popping up all around you. The slang term is named after a German terrorist group known as the Baader-Meinhof gang, because a newspaper commentator noticed the name of the ultra-left German terrorist group two times in twenty-four hours. The phrase "Baader-Meinhof phenomenon" became a meme in the mid-1990s.

When I graduated from my CERT training course, I started noticing more situations where I could be useful. The skills I learned in class gave me the confidence to offer assistance. I witnessed Citi bike accidents, homeless people shivering and in need, playground accidents in the park. My training opened my eyes to situations where my new skill set could be useful. It was my version of the Baader-Meinhof phenomenon.

I delivered blankets and warm clothing to the homeless. During a hurricane, we checked on our elderly neighbors when we lost power. We collected food and baby formula, diapers and water. When a gas line exploded and scores of families were left without a home, we did a clothing drive. When it snowed, I rushed outside to measure the drifts so the Office of Emergency Management would have accurate information from all around the city. I did community outreach and taught classes on how to prepare a "go bag." This is a portable satchel of necessities, including food, water, and medicine to last one person three days. At the time, I was writing a weekly online column for the *New York Daily News*, and I used that and my social media to communicate with my fellow New Yorkers about emergency preparation.

The night of our final CERT certification examination was the same night as the Metropolitan Museum Costume Institute Ball. The theme for the gala was Super Heroes, which seemed fitting in light of how we viewed our first responder teachers. My buddy and former Batman George Clooney was one of the hosts. The event is a hot ticket, but I needed to fulfill my obligation to my CERT team. I also did not want to miss what would be one wild party. I took my final exam in a voluminous off the shoulder formal ball gown. I hiked up my skirt and demonstrated my newly honed CPR skills. I don't remember explaining why I was taking the test in formal wear, and I don't recall anyone asking. Maybe they thought I was dolled up to get a better grade? I passed the test and then celebrated like an unsupervised teenager at the Met Ball after-party.

Not long after I passed my course and became an active member of Manhattan Community Board Number Two Community Emergency Response Team, I witnessed a traffic accident on my corner. A cab had hit an elderly gentleman who was crossing the street. One of the first things I learned in training was to secure the location. I immediately called 911 and then had the cab driver get out and direct traffic so the victim wouldn't get run over again while he was lying in the street.

Then I tended to the accident victim. He was conscious, so I introduced myself and asked his name.

"Ivan," he replied.

"Ivan, can I sit with you until the ambulance arrives?"

"Ambulance? What's wrong with me?"

THINGS TO SAY IN AN EMERGENCY

- There, there
- It's all okay
- You'll be fine
- I'm here for you
- I find that when I am scared, having sex usually cheers me right up (use at your discretion)

THINGS NOT TO SAY IN AN EMERGENCY

- Calm down!
- Stop your pathetic whining
- I can see the white meat
- Oh my God, it's a bloodbath!
- THE HORROR! THE HORROR!

I could see that Ivan was bleeding from a head wound, but I was a rookie, and I thought the best thing to do was fudge the truth. I took his hand and tried to comfort him. I didn't want to tell him about the blood. I didn't want to panic him. So I told him he was fine and I was going to sit with him.

I may have overdone the comforting, because he replied, "Well, if I'm okay, I'll just get up." Our training had stressed that if the victim was in a safe place, we were not to move them. So I kept telling Ivan to just stay put, and Ivan kept trying to get up. Finally I told him that I was a trained Community Emergency Response Team Volunteer and ordered him to stay still or I'd sit on him. He still didn't listen. So I sat on him, until the paramedics got there and asked me what the hell I was doing sitting on an accident victim.

It wasn't a textbook example of how to handle an emergency. But I'd assessed the situation, made priorities, formulated a plan, and put it into action, just as John Leach described.

- -

CPR

Everyone should know how to do CPR, because it really can save lives. But few people know how to do it, and it's easy to do it wrong. If I ever got a tattoo, I would have a CPR how-to list tattooed on my chest. In case I keeled over from a heart attack, a passing Good Samaritan could just follow the instructions. Meanwhile, here's a clip-and-save list you can carry in your purse or wallet, courtesy of the Red Cross.

For an adult who does not demonstrate signs of life, begin CPR using the following steps:

- Open airway and give two rescue breaths
- Compress chest thirty times
- Give two rescue breaths
- Compress chest thirty times
- Continue cycles of two breaths and thirty compressions

There's also hands-only CPR, which is just chest compression. You can see it demonstrated here:

https://www.youtube.com/watch?v=n5hP4DIBCEE

Either way, remember to compress the chest approximately 120 times a minute. Conveniently, this is the same as the beat to the song "Stayin' Alive." Don't stop pumping until the paramedics show up!

- -

FIRST AID MNEMONICS

The more people who learn first aid and know what to do in an emergency, the better we are as a society. We will have better prepared people and more skillful citizens on public transportation, in schools, at stadiums, and just walking down the street.

If your brain is anything like mine, it's probably filled with useless things like the theme songs to long-canceled TV shows. Why not delete the lyrics to the *Love Boat* theme song and replace them with something useful, like these first aid mnemonics?

A mnemonic is a pattern of letters or words used to help with memorization. The word comes from the Greek goddess of memory, Mnemosyne.

These mnemonics will help you recall the proper emergency first aid actions that could keep a person alive until the EMTs arrive:

- PEEP (for a major bleeding wound): Position person on the floor, Expose wound, Elevate injury, apply Pressure
- PULSE (signs of a heart attack): Persistent chest pain, Upset stomach, Lightheadedness, Shortness of breath, Excessive swaying. Always carry a baby aspirin with you—if you have these symptoms and take a baby aspirin, you could save your life.
- To treat shock: Face is red, raise the head. Face is pale, raise the tail.
- RICE (for a sprain or strain): Rest, Ice, Comfortable position/Compression, Elevation

- PLASTIC (signs and symptoms of a fracture): Pain, Loss of movement, Angulation, Swelling, Tenderness, Irregularity, Crepitus (popping or crackling noises)

- -

- -

YOUR GO BAG

A "go bag" is a collection of items you may need in case of an emergency. You may have to evacuate, though most people never will—it's more likely you'll need to "shelter in place," or stay where you are. No matter what situation arises, every person in the house should have a "go bag" stocked and readily accessible, including pets and in-laws. The best option is a backpack, which will leave your hands free so you can hold a flashlight or a cell phone and the hand of a loved one. A backpack on wheels or a rolling suitcase is a good alternative.

Your "go bag" should contain:

- Enough food, water, and medicine for three days. These are the most important things.
- Copies of your important documents in a waterproof ziplock bag. (Insurance cards, ID, proof of address, special family photos, etc.)
- Extra house and car keys.
- Credit and ATM cards.
- Cash in small denominations—at least fifty to one hundred dollars.
- Flashlight and batteries. (LED flashlights are more durable and last ten times longer than traditional flashlights.)

- A manual hand-cranked radio or battery-operated radio. Manual radios often have cell phone charging features, solar power options, flashlight, siren, and compass.
- A list of medications for each family member, why they take it, and the dosage.
- Sharpie marker so you can write names and contact information on the arm of a kid, or an elderly or non-verbal person.
- Extra eyeglasses.
- First aid kit.
- Waterproof matches, Swiss army knife, rain ponchos, thermal blankets, extra socks and underwear.
- Hygiene items.
- Childcare items.
- Small map of the region.
- Small personal comfort items or games, like playing cards.

- -

FIRST AID MNEMONIC CARD

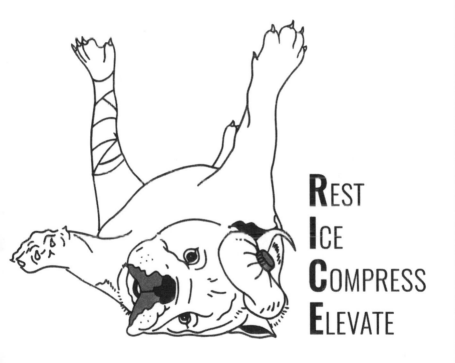

REST
ICE
COMPRESS
ELEVATE

UN COUPLE MALADE: THE RELATIONSHIP BETWEEN DOCTOR AND PATIENT

DE CLERAMBAULT'S SYNDROME IS an amorous delusion in which the stricken person incorrectly believes that an exalted person is in love with her. The object of the delusion is usually older and of a higher social status; quite often, the focus of de Clerambault's syndrome is the patient's doctor. The relationship is entirely imaginary on the part of the patient. Dr. Gaetan de Clerambault was a highly regarded French doctor and artist who first described his experience of patients with the syndrome that now bears his name. He called it Psychose Passionelle; it's now more widely known as erotomania, where romantic feelings are targeted toward a powerful person. Sigmund Freud called the misinterpretation of bedside manner "transference." The Florence Nightingale effect is the opposite, a syndrome in which a caregiver develops romantic feelings for a patient who does not return the affection.

I don't have de Clerambault's Syndrome, aka Psychose Passionelle, nor have I been the object of a caregiver's Florence Nightingale Effect, but I will cop to being part of a different kind of disease romance. I'm part of "un couple malade"—a

French phrase that translates to "a wedding made in illness." I adore my neurologist, Dr. Frank Petito, who guides me and advises me on how to live my best life while managing a rare and incurable illness. He's got all the qualities of a wonderful, caring partner. I jumped onto his coattails, and I've been hanging on for dear life ever since. I may not have de Clerambault's Syndrome, but when medical science finds a cure for sarcoidosis, I'll need to go into treatment for Stockholm syndrome. I identify as Dr. Petito's patient as much as I do as a wife and hockey mom.

The medical system can be wildly intimidating, and I realized very early on that if I wanted to improve my medical condition, I needed to be more than an unlucky passive observer of my illness and my treatment. When I first became symptomatic, I consulted my general practitioner, Dr. Matarese. He stayed late in his office to give me a checkup. He saw I was weak, in pain, and in bad shape. He asked me to wait while he called the hospital to schedule a battery of neurological tests for the next morning. He was direct and comforting, and the last thing he said to me was, "I don't know what this is, and I'm not going to sugarcoat it. You may have a very serious illness and you need to stay strong and keep a level head. Stay vigilant and beware of charlatans. There are people who will try to take advantage of a sick person's desire to get better, so be careful who you listen to when it comes to your treatment." I send Dr. Matarese a thank-you note every year for the advice he gave me on that memorable September night.

Your relationship with your doctor is intimate. He's going to assist you with monumental decisions about your body. Your doctor will see you naked and weak and at your worst. He'll know your *real* weight, not your driver's license weight. He'll ask you about your bathroom habits, and he'll know which style of bikini wax you're sporting, and whether you let your landing strip expand into the Jimi-Hendrix-is-giving-me-a-piggy-back-style.

The medical system can be incredibly dehumanizing. Part of it is that there are so many sick people. The system is not designed to soothe your feelings, and doctors often become desensitized. They see a lot of suffering, and the average length of an office visit is about fifteen minutes. You can prepare for your visits by showing up on time, even though you know he'll keep you waiting. Instead of pacing the waiting room like a silverback gorilla, write down questions you might forget and review your notes. Even when you find the right doctor, you've still got to do some heavy lifting in the relationship.

Communication is the key to making a doctor-patient relationship work. A lot of our medical decisions will be made in a crisis frame of mind. So we rely on the expertise of our doctor to guide us to the right choice. Healthcare is too often a blind purchase, a matter of choosing someone from a list provided by your insurance carrier. When you are chronically ill, you have to look a lot harder to find the doctor who is right for you; someone who can act as your team captain and communicate with all your other doctors. You wouldn't marry someone on the basis of a Tinder profile, right? I mean, not until you had sex with them first.

It took many months to find a doctor who possessed the optimism and fearless pharmacology I needed. My nerve pain and respiratory issues were hard to manage before I met Dr. Petito, but the wait was worth it. I made an immediate connection with him, and I felt right away that we'd make a good team. Dr. Frank Petito is a national treasure. He's one of the top neurologists in the world. He treats the heads of heads of state as well as my own ordinary melon.

I've been a chronic patient for fifteen years now, and my relationship with my doctor has progressed. We've been together longer than my husband and I have been married. In the way I like to shower my husband with unusual tokens of appreciation such as antique medical devices and wooden legs, Dr. Petito's presents are also medically inspired. He travels to his office at the hospital via a vintage light blue girl's three-speed bike, and for a long time he didn't wear a helmet. The smartest man in the world when it comes to the brain refused to wear a brain bucket! I was concerned that his gray matter remain intact so it could keep on taking care of my gray matter, so I commissioned an artist to paint a proper bike safety helmet with anatomically correct right and left hemispheres.

I'd say I'm getting good value out of the gifts. I gave him pewter cufflinks that show the lower digestive system at work, and he gave me a way to live a big beautiful life with sarcoidosis. I can't imagine being sick without Dr. Petito. If they ever find a cure for sarcoidosis, I would keep going to appointments and showing up with crackpot gewgaws, like a reflex hammer in the shape of a giant Viagra pill.

Not long ago, a young woman I mentor invited me to a lunch at her apartment, and I noticed that the hand holding her iced tea had a slight tremor. I am hypersensitive to neurological symptoms, and I had a feeling something was up, but I respected her privacy; I didn't pry.

A few weeks later, she called and said, "We need to talk." I had a feeling it was serious, so I took her out to lunch. We went to the Soho House for the second-best burger in NYC. It turned out that this slim, gorgeous woman could beat Joey

Chestnutt in any competitive eating contest. After she ate all of my French fries, she confided that she had a brain tumor and was about to begin a course of radiation at Memorial Sloan Kettering hospital.

I had anticipated she was going to share bad news, and I came prepared. I had ordered a box of three hundred candy necklaces as a present for her. "Hand them out to everyone you see at the hospital," I told her. "Doctors, nurses, technicians, other patients, little kids, the security guard . . . whomever you see and whenever the feeling moves you. Everyone likes a present, and when you give something away, it takes away the focus off of your problems. You share a small bit of happiness with a stranger."

My pal filled her purse with the candy necklaces and handed them out as instructed. The reaction was so encouraging, she upped the ante and beat me at my own game. She bought shocking pink lipstick for all her nurses. She is very convincing and encouraged all of the nurses, women and men, to trust her and try it on. I love the image of the Schiaparelli pink-lipped smiles on the no-nonsense nurses of the oncology unit. The makeup didn't make up for the fact she was going through a difficult time, but it shifted the focus and brought some happiness and glamour to the hospital.

A successful couple malade is one in which the doctor encourages the patient to advocate for herself and use her own powers of courage, tenacity, humor, and acceptance to find a way to coexist with her disease. You don't have to bribe your way to a better healthcare experience with candy necklaces or Viagra reflex hammers. You don't have to joke around like it's open mic night at the Chuckle Factory. You don't have to engage in conversation—just be polite and hold the door. If you are going to the water cooler, ask the person near you if you can get them a paper cone of water as well. You can improve your experience by making a conscious effort to do a small gesture of kindness toward yourself, your fellow patients, and your medical team.

I average about an operation every other year, and before I go under the knife, I write messages on my body for my surgeon. Notes like "thanks for operating on me," "make sure you get the right side," and "are you single? If so, have I got a hot guy for you."

A hospital is no place for a sick person. You are already suffering, and now you fend off continuing assaults on your person, your dignity, and your immune system. It is stressful. It is noisy. The food is lousy, and the decor is worse. Just when you need privacy to reflect and gather the courage to deal with your visiting in-laws, you are subjected to an intrusion about your bathroom habits. I think a useful equation is for every day you spend in the chaotic atmosphere of hospital, you need to spend two days at home recovering.

A relationship is constant work. You're always in it. The same is true for being a part of un couple malade. I'm not with my husband all the time, and I can go for weeks without seeing my doctor. But my illness never ends, and neither do my interactions with the medical system. I've been having some scary vision problems, and I have a stellar ophthalmologist. He told me that since I am a compliant patient, he felt comfortable monitoring my symptoms before launching into an aggressive treatment plan. When the time came for treatment, he prescribed eye medication. Before I put these drops in my eyes, I hold the bottle in my hand and take a moment to be grateful. I'm appreciative that when I was in college going out to the campus Rathskeller on Twofer Tuesdays Ladies Night,

Dr. Belgorade was studying in the lab and learning how to one day save my vision. He doesn't know I say a prayer of thanks, any more than my husband knows the silent prayer of thanks I say every day for having met him. Respect and gratitude are keys to a successful marriage and to a successful couple malade.

I'm also grateful for the pharmacists who compound and dispense the medicines that calm my seizures, help dull my nerve pain, and may save my vision. I'm grateful to Julio, the guy from the pharmacy who delivers my medications, but I get to deliver my thanks to him in a more concrete way. The other day he told me he's thinking about getting on Tinder to find a steady girlfriend. "Not with that haircut, my friend," I told him. I think he was grateful to me, because he got a great-looking haircut, although not a girlfriend yet.

But not every marriage was made to last forever. If your doctor isn't holding up her end of the deal, it may be time to move on and look for a new medical relationship. It can be hard to "break up" with your doctor, so I created a form to make it easier. You can fill it out and mail it to your physician to spare yourself the extra stress of "It's not me, it is *you*" conversation. Just take it from me, don't get schnockered and text your ex-doctor at 4:00 a.m. Nothing good will come of it.

My husband is staggeringly healthy. He rowed crew and played soccer in school. He gets up at 5:30 a.m. to go to spin class. He does yoga. He never gets a cold. He recently got a standing desk, and somehow got a hernia out of it. He had no interest in developing his own couple malade. He was having none of it. "I just want to get it over with," he said.

I took him to the hospital early in the morning. After his surgery, the nurses let me into the recovery room. He was hopped up on goofballs and still woozy from the anesthesia.

I thought it would be fun to tease him and tell him that the recovery room was purgatory and I just saw his recently deceased grandmother, who was waiting for him. He was groggy as hell, but he saw through that pretty quickly. Then I tried to convince him that he had not had his surgery yet. I was just getting started, but at this point the attending nurse threw me out of the room. You would think I'd be more compassionate, but sometimes I'm better at being part of the doctor-patient relationship than the regular kind.

- -

BREAK UP WITH YOUR DOCTOR NOTE

Dear Dr. _____,

It's been great being your patient, and we've had a good run. You kept me from dying, which is something I'll always treasure. And I'll never forget the day you _____ my _____. Who could?

But recently I feel like we've grown apart. _____ at your office just don't give me the same excitement they used to. And I know you're feeling the same thing.

For both our sakes, I think it's time to move on. I'll find another doctor; you'll find other patients. It's better this way, and I think we'll both be happier.

With hopes of good health,

_____

P.S. I will be unfollowing you on all social media.

- -

BITE THE BULLET BADGE

You earned it!

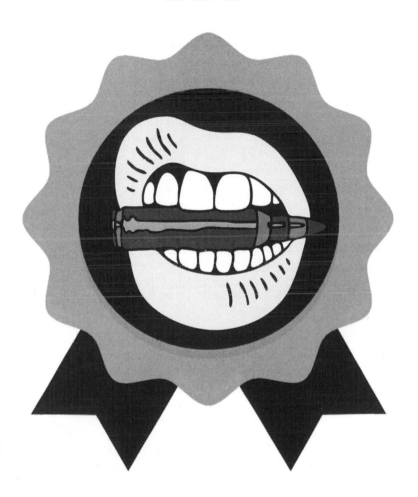

BIBLIOTHERAPY:
READ TWO BOOKS AND
CALL ME IN THE MORNING

Jean Anthelme Brillat-Savarin, French gourmand and epicurean, wrote, "Tell me what you eat and I will tell you what you are." We are what we consume, and I believe this applies both inside and outside of the digestive system. Brillat-Savarin's quote also applies to reading: Tell me what you read, and I'll tell you who you are.

Who I am changes with the unpredictable flares and the progressive, degenerative effects of my illness. I can't foresee what level of pain I'll have when I wake up. Some days I am high functioning, other days I'm cooped up at home because air hurts my skin. On better days, I work, I see friends, I cook nice dinners, and I incorporate long walks into my routine. On the days I'm housebound and can't do a lot because of the pain and the effects of powerful medication, I do research, take Internet courses, and write letters. On days I can't even do a little, I order in food, hole up in my couch fort, and read.

Reading has been a great source of happiness and contentment. I recall the moment I became literate: my dad taught me to read with the book *Hop on Pop*. From then on, I'd wall myself off from my siblings and read the backs of all the cereal boxes at the breakfast table. I'd even read the hallmark on the spoons we used to shovel Cap'n Crunch into our masticating maws. The library is as sacred as a church to me, and the annual book sale, where I fill bags of books for one dollar a pop, is like Christmas. I read to be less stupid; as Caitlyn Moran wrote, I "read myself a new brain."

I always have a book in my pocket or my bag, and a stack on my bedside table. Every horizontal surface is jammed with books. I have piles on the floor. I need books like a vampire needs blood. As Oscar Wilde wrote, "It's what you read when you don't have to that determines what you will be when you can't help it." I read to get lost in a story, and to find myself on the page.

Reading is being studied as a way to deal with chronic pain. Researchers at the University of Liverpool have noted that reading and cognitive behavioral therapy have similar effects on the brain. Reading can trigger positive memories as the reader becomes engaged in the book. The investment in a story or poem triggers the recall of positive memories and sends new pain-free messages to the brain. The study didn't share titles of books, but I would steer clear of *Old Yeller* and *Sounder* or any of the other puppy snuff books I read as a kid. I am still traumatized.

My primary complementary therapy for pain is reading. I use books to distract myself from pain flares. I have my faith, my personal experience, and science backing me up that distraction is one of the most highly endorsed and most commonly used strategies for relief. By directing your focus on another processing activity, it is possible to perceive less pain. The mental distraction of reading words on a page can actually inhibit incoming pain signals.

I take my prescribed medication in exact measurements at exact times. My compliance with my pharmaceuticals is the most disciplined segment of my life. But I am immoderate with reading. I am happiest with my head in a book, tea in my favorite cup, and Sinatra, Van Morrison, or Herb Alpert in my ears. I will read multiple books at once. I'll start from the last page and read a book backwards and I will read into the wee small hours until my eyes feel scratchy. Then I squeeze out some eye drops and keep reading. My husband will kiss me goodnight before he goes to sleep, and when he wakes up I'll still be on the chaise, where he saw me eight hours ago, reading a new book. My Kindle is my electronic opiate. I read with the relentlessness of a compulsive gambler betting on the ponies.

I hate to shop, except for books. Because I'm a Cheap Pete, used bookstores are irresistible to me. I live a few blocks from the Strand Bookstore, a New York City landmark with over six miles of books in the stacks. I visit the Strand more than I visit the grocery store.

One night, walking home from dinner with my pal Vig, I decided to pop into the Strand before it closed. I was up on the third floor checking out some art books when I heard a commotion. I looked across the room and saw a disheveled man on the staircase, brandishing a huge piece of lumber. He was screaming and whirling his very intimidating makeshift javelin.

It was pretty clear that no one was going to go up or down the stairs, and sure enough, he shouted, "No one is going up or down these stairs." I wasn't going to argue. He was either on drugs, was having a psychotic episode, or both.

At this point, my Community Emergency Response Team training kicked in. One of the first things you learn is stay safe, so I decided the safest place to cower in fear was next to the burliest cashier. I hid behind the counter, and my new cashier friend said the police had been called and were on their way. I asked him if this happened often and would he judge me if I wet my pants in fear. He was not fazed and was the very picture of a bored bookstore clerk. I imagine this might not have been his first psychotic lance wielder. He said it would all be over soon.

Soon could not come fast enough. To distract myself from the floor show, I picked up a book that was underneath the counter. It was an author-signed copy of *Ota Benga: The Pygmy in the Zoo* by Phillips Verner Bradford and Harvey Blume. To read about a fellow human being exhibited in my city's largest zoo, just a little bit more than a century ago, was a revolting and distressing discovery.

The EMTs and police officers arrived and bravely handled the man on the staircase. We were invited to leave, but reading about the tragic, brutal, and incomprehensible life of Ota Benga rooted me in place until closing time at 10:30 p.m. (Yes, I bought the book.)

Astronomer Galileo Galilei wrote that reading is almost like a superpower in its ability to connect us with distant peoples and places that we may never see in life. Recent studies have confirmed his insight. In a study described in the *Annual Review of Psychology*, when subjects read about other people's experiences in a book, it activated the same regions of their brains as if they had experienced the event themselves. Books transport us and give us access to experiences we will never have. Ota Benga's biography transported me from twenty-first-century Greenwich Village to the Belgian Congo and back to the early twentieth century Bronx. Books, according to the study, are like embalmed brains.

Bibliotherapy is the practice of reading books with the goal of ameliorating or even resolving emotional issues. Reading relieves stress and has been shown to lower blood pressure. Bibliotherapy has been proven to comfort patients with depression and insomnia, which are the evil stepsisters of chronic pain. Chronic illness and chronic pain are isolating. Why not use the time alone to crack open a book? Books give us a place to go when we are stuck in bed. Reading makes us smarter and more empathetic. The positive physical and psychological effects of reading may help us live longer. Or, if the book is slow, life will just feel longer.

Bibliotherapy can be practiced with literature, novels, nonfiction, poetry, philosophy . . . it's your call. Books heighten your knowledge and analytical skills. Philosopher John Locke wrote, "Reading furnishes the mind only with materials of knowledge: it is the thinking that makes what we read ours." Reading gives your brain a workout, engages concentration, and slows down age-related dementia. Hell, you can even burn calories while reading. If you sit up while reading, you burn about seventy to ninety calories an hour . . . about the equivalent of a glass of white wine. Which sounds nice right about now, doesn't it?

Bibliotherapy is an ancient practice. Reading novels is not a novel cure. Literature can illuminate what is possible for us. Hope is imagining better possibilities; a reminder that something exists that is bigger and better than the challenges and pains of daily life. The motto A House of Healing for the Soul was inscribed about the entrance of the royal library in Thebes, Egypt, in about 150 BC. (This was when books were written on rolls of papyrus. Just try to dog-ear your place on a scroll.) The ancients knew that reading was one way to calm and inspire a stressed mind. More recently, soldiers returning home from the battlefields of World War I were prescribed a syllabus of good books to help them process the trauma of war. Sigmund Freud used literature during psychoanalysis.

In the 1400s, most of the population of Western Europe could not read. And even if they could, there were very few books available. Before the invention of the printing press, a group of scribes in the Middle Ages could spend years creating a book. They were hunched over their ergonomically incorrect copy tables risking carpal tunnel syndrome and weakened eyesight from the strain. They wrote next to the chill of drafty windows, as the risk of a candle igniting the paper was too great.

It was a strenuous and momentous task. Books were treasured valuables, and scribes would write curses in the front of the book, threatening pain and suffering to thieves and anyone who dog-eared a page. "Whoever steals this book, let him die the death: let him be frizzled with pain, may the falling sickness rage within him. May he be broken on the wheel or hanged," runs one especially vivid book curse. Be sure to return your borrowed books.

The Gutenberg press liberated the printed word (and the scribes) and democratized knowledge. Philosopher Marshall McLuhan said that practically every aspect of modern life is a direct consequence of the printing press, and despite the rise of e-book readers, I agree. A good rule of thumb is that if you feel that you have not read enough, you haven't read enough.

Reading is a pathway to the essence of who you are. Groucho Marx, whose collection of letters is one of my favorite books, said, "Outside of a dog, a book is man's best friend. Inside of a dog, it's too dark to read." Trust me—I'm a professional emeritus therapeutic recreational specialist, hospital chaplain, certified civilian community responder, and now an armchair bibliotherapist.

BIBLIOMANCY

Bibliomancy is a form of divination, using books to answer questions or get advice or insight. The practice of using a book to tell the future is as old as books themselves. It's probably even older, as Torah scrolls were sometimes used for the purpose. The method is simple: pick a book, most often a bible or a philosophy book, but any kind of book will do. Close your eyes and let the book fall open, then put your finger on a page. Read the word or phrase you've selected (you can pry your open your eyes for this part) and, so the belief states, it will give you the answer you seek.

BIBLIOTHERAPY BRAIN

Read yourself a new brain!

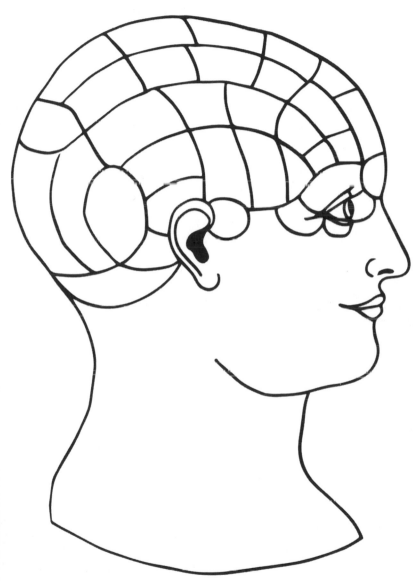

Write down the titles of the books you read in the segments in the head. Fill up your brain with 33 new books.

THE NON-MONUMENTAL THEORY OF HAPPINESS

HAPPINESS IS NOT A perfect life. No one has that. A happy life is not about the monumental moments of good fortune, like hitting the lotto, winning the Stanley Cup, or a tequila-fueled night with Brad Pitt. Those things are great, and congratulations if they happen to you. But they don't have staying power. The French writer, polymath, and bon vivant Bernard de Fontanelle wrote that "a great obstacle to happiness is to expect too much happiness." I would add that another hurdle to happiness is putting too much stock in the rare yet monumental events of life to make us happy. Our happiness is not in the greatest hits; it's not in the fanfare—it is found in the small moments in between.

You don't have to try to be happy when bad things happen to a good egg like you. It can be incredibly difficult to be cheery or even content when you are coexisting with chronic pain. It can feel like there is no space to breathe and that whatever good thing might happen is nowhere enough to compensate for the overwhelming presence of pain and disease. Whoever said "No pain, no gain," I bet didn't live in chronic pain.

Don't let a pain flare or a bad day trick you into thinking that you have a bad life. It is possible to be content and be in catastrophic knuckle-dragging pain at the same time. There is always space and possibility for happiness. As the religious author Charles R. Swindoll wrote, "I am convinced that life is 10 percent what happens to me and 90 percent of how I react to it. And so it is with you. We are in charge of our attitudes."

Studies show that 50 percent of your happiness level is innate, which seems daunting—half of our happiness level is preset! I am a happiness-level-half-full kind of gal. I do believe we can increase our happiness, and science confirms that we can alter our brains to let more happiness in. The question is, how?

Philosopher Arthur Schopenhauer believed that happiness is the absence of suffering. I believe happiness is the presence of gratitude, even in the presence of suffering. Our history is written by people who have suffered and gone on to live accomplished and fulfilled lives. C. S. Lewis advised, "Don't let your happiness depend on something you may lose." My view is that happiness arises from looking beyond imperfections and pain and focusing on the small, inspiring daily occurrences that give us pleasure. The little joys of our ordinary life. It's the sum of our everyday conventional acts of small kindness that add up to greater happiness. A friendly greeting to the corner fruit vendor, collecting the mail for your elderly neighbor, giving the homeless woman on the street a bottle of water on a hot day—these minor moments add up to a major sense of well being. Our gratitude for the little joys in life can increase our baseline happiness. It is not the extraordinary strokes of good fortune; it's the pleasing, ordinary daily exchanges. I call this the "Non-Monumental Exchange Theory of Happiness."

I'm going through a monumentally distressing deterioration right now. I'm having trouble with my eyes, and I now need surgery. I just saw Dr. Petito, my neurologist and my rock, and I was on the verge of losing it. I wasn't crying, but my eyes were swimming with tears. He commented, "You're usually so stoic. You're my toughest patient. I've never seen you like this." I replied, "You don't know what it's like. I've been getting a surgery every other year. I'm losing parts of my body. It's a lot."

I'll probably need some help walking again. I was surveying my umbrella stand full of canes, and I realized I was uncertain about going out in public using one again. I felt like a fraud with my cane. I felt like a dandy or a fop, an impersonation of my usual scrappy self.

I cannot stop the progressive deterioration of my disease. This is out of my control. I can only control how I feel about the loss. My toes are taped together inside my shoes, the buddy system to keep them in line. The fingers on my left hand are more like vestigial tails than working flexible digits. In the glory days, when I was riding the express elevator to the penthouse overlooking Success Street and could take in the view with two eyes, I considered myself an appreciative person. But is it possible that I am even more grateful because I've had so much and then lost so much?

I'm counting my blessings and grateful that someone has held the door for me. As I step over the threshold, I'm grateful they didn't trip me. It makes me satisfied and happy just to walk around my neighborhood. I look forward to the banter with Mohammad, the corner fruit vendor, and how the other Mohammad at the coffee cart makes my cup just the way I like it . . . lots of milk, no sugar. These are not big events. These are the ordinary moments of everyday life. I can focus my thoughts on feeling gratitude for the day. I am cognizant of the small, non-monumental moments that give life to my life.

Every day we have a choice, to be useless or useful. I find it's nearly impossible to feel sad or sorry for myself if I'm being of service. If you have done no good for others, you have not done anything great. Happiness doesn't spring from what we get; it arises from what we give. Happiness is a byproduct of being useful. Goethe said, "Knowing is not enough, we must apply. Wishing is not enough, we must do."

My theory of the Non-Monumental Exchange grew from my experience with illness. On one hand, I have a lot of what you could call ill fortune. I lost my good health, my fertility, and my former career in broadcasting. But rather than waiting for a massive bit of good luck to cheer me up, I made my own luck. I magnified my appreciation for small things. A walk along the Hudson River on a beautiful morning can make my day. When I'm not balled up in pain, I stretch out and do a jig in appreciation of the reprieve. I learned to fly when the window is open.

Adversity can create an opportunity for self-discovery. When you are faced with an ongoing medical catastrophe, it forces you to take notice of the little things that you might have overlooked when you were dazzled by good health. You recognize that the little moments are not so little. The appreciation of accumulated small moments can create a happier life. Novelist George Eliot captured this perfectly when she wrote, "the growing good of the world is partly dependent on unhistoric acts."

Life is more than breath and a heartbeat. It is about meaning and purpose. It is about who you become and what you contribute. Who you are will be measured by what you did in your daily life. You only get one life, so you'd best do what you can to grasp the happiness available to you. A mosaic is made up of thousands of small, shiny, broken fragments. I believe that when we face obstacles and adversity in our lives, we have an opportunity to strengthen our courage. Victor Frankl wrote, "If there is meaning in life at all, then there must be meaning in suffering."

The pursuit of happiness is not a selfish endeavor. Thomas Jefferson cited happiness as one of our unalienable rights in the US Declaration of Independence, because happiness has tangible benefits. Happy people are more productive and motivated. Happy people build on happiness every day. Each small act of kindness and generosity has a positive effect. Even with the smallest gesture, like giving a friendly wave rather than the finger when you get cut off on the highway, you can create peace instead of confrontation.

There are days when it seems like nothing good is coming your way. A bad day does not equal a bad life. But those days can feel much worse when you're already enduring a chronic condition. It's raining, your joints ache, you feel as weak as a kitten. Then, your phone fell in the toilet and you outgrew your fat pants.

When I have days like this, I think of the motto my family believes in: "Life gives to the giver and takes from the taker." Even though the toilet took my phone, I can give my fat pants to Goodwill. It is up to me to save myself. It is my responsibility to see what good I can rescue from a bad day. Be miserable, or motivate myself. It's my choice.

I like to write letters thanking people who have inspired me, but some days the damage in my left ulnar nerve causes pain so intensely sharp I cannot hold a pen. I can still practice gratitude.

It takes nothing besides the consciousness to be grateful. If I can't be grateful for today, I will rewind gratitude for something that happened yesterday. Something non-monumental, like a joke my husband told me, or witnessing the kindness of the visiting nurses toward my neighbor, who has Parkinson's disease. Or I could be grateful for something that didn't happen ... and appreciate that I didn't grow an Amish man's beard overnight from the prednisone. Or that Carvel has not discontinued the Cookie Puss ice cream cake, our family's go-to celebration dessert. That makes me monumentally happy.

It seems that things turn out for the best for those who try and make the best of their situation. It is a mistake to do nothing, just because there are days I can only do a little. If I were productive only on days I felt well, I would never do anything. The way to get big things done is to start with small actions and keep doing them. These minor successive changes can add up to major accomplishments and improvements in your happiness.

- -

THE KAREN DUFFY NO-STRESS TEST

The Holmes and Rahe Stress Test is self-assessment tool that helps you understand the total burden of stress in your life. The higher the score, the more likely you are to become ill in the next three years. And while it's important to know the negative stressors, I think it's a good counterpoint to measure the small joys in your life. Each event below has a number attached; add up the points for everything that happened to you today, and then see the assessment at the end.

No-Stress Test:

Good hair day: 5 points
Good head day (if bald): 5 points
Someone noticed your good hair: 10 points
Found a great hat to cover your bad hair day: 10
Complimented someone else's hair: 15 points
Excellent medical checkup: 10 points
In-laws moved far, far away: 100 points
In-laws moved to a place with no cell service: 500 points
Found money on the street: 5 points
Leftover Cookie Puss in freezer: 15 points
Didn't grow lady mustache from steroids: 25 points
Still fit in your fat pants: 10 points
Scale broke—error in your favor: 15 points
Best friend declared it's the beginning of bourbon season
    and poured out two fingers of Maker's Mark: 50 points
Won a taxidermy skunk in eBay auction: 20 points
Son made you a sandwich*: 30 points
Helper monkey made dinner*: 100 points
Son learned how to make dinner*: 250 points

------

* Have you noticed that food tastes better when someone else makes it,
even when it's just a sandwich, even when it's a sandwich made by a helper
monkey? There's a scientific reason. Researchers at Carnegie Mellon found
that when you cook for yourself, you experience the sight, smell, and tex-
tures of the food during the prep. You've "pre-consumed" it. The extended
stimulus makes eating the food less novel and less desirable. When someone else makes food for you, all the sensations are a surprise, and you enjoy
them more.

How to evaluate your score:

The higher the better, but anything above a zero is great. You have enough stress in your life. To your final score you can add a bonus of one hundred points for just taking the test. If that doesn't make you happy, well, I don't even know.

- -

—I'M USING THIS CARD TO—

DUFF OUT

I CAN'T TODAY

• TALK AT YOUR OWN RISK •

THE UPSIDE OF A LIFE
TURNED UPSIDE DOWN

THE OBSTACLES WE FACE can impede us or they can inspire us. As C. S. Lewis wrote, "Hardships often prepare ordinary people for an extraordinary destiny." Pain and illness can't take away the things that really matter: self-respect, gratitude, and resilience. Life is more than brain waves, heartbeats, and breaths. Finding your purpose and giving and receiving love gives *life* to our lives. We have the power to define what our lives mean; we are the architects of our future.

I would not wish a life with chronic pain on my worst enemy. A painful life-altering event is one of the top fears for most of the population. We who are chronically ill deal with what most people fear every single day. We know our complaints are not moral weaknesses. We find resilience, we adapt, and we figure out a new way to live. We have guts.

We look for meaning in a life colored by pain, suffering, and obstacles. Our struggles teach us skills to overcome them. Our closeness to death can give our lives urgency. Our suffering illuminates who we are.

I don't miss my old life because I don't remember it. I've forgotten what it feels like to not live in unrelenting pain. I have found a new way to live with a purpose.

On about half of my days, pain flares have me housebound. There is an unpredictability that comes from a chronic condition. It creates instability. Poet John Keats used the phrase "negative capability," meaning "the willingness to embrace uncertainty, live with mystery and make peace with ambiguity." I cannot control when the pain flares tether me to my home, roped to my bed like Gulliver. I can only control how I will react. I have no choice but to suck it up and accept it.

When you live with a chronic illness, an upside is acceptance. It doesn't mean resignation. I still have hope that my pain will diminish. Acceptance is understanding the challenges we face and making peace with these obstacles. I have room in my life where pain and hope are compatible. Resilience is finding a way to coexist with our trials. It's the ability to deal with setbacks, crises, and pain with courage. It's the quality that keeps me from giving up. Recognize all you have to be thankful for, as this fosters resilience. It is never too late to get smarter. I won't let the obstacles of relentless pain and illness capsize my life.

The progressive nature of a degenerative illness has magnified my appreciation for life. In the twelfth century, the Persian poet Rumi wrote, "The wound is the place where the light enters you." If I hated my disease, I would hate a big part of my life. I want to keep letting the light in.

Acceptance unleashes me from the resentment that life didn't turn out the way I expected. My illness doesn't limit my enthusiasm for life, but it rattles my cage every day. It's frustrating to lose my motor skills, the simple ability to open a door, tie my shoes, or write legibly. So I wear slip-on loafers and use tape to attach the pen to my fingers and thumb. I've had so many pain flares that I've milked two books and countless articles out of them. I am challenged and discouraged by my setbacks. But I learned that failure is temporary, and giving up is forever. Theodore Roosevelt wrote that "it is only through labor and painful effort, by grim energy and resolute courage, that we move on to better things."

In the early phase of my illness, I was embarrassed by the deficits caused by my disease. I was ashamed, the way you would feel self-conscious and try to hide a big ugly stain on the back of your dress. I've learned to shed embarrassment and focus on acceptance. Now it is impossible for me to feel ashamed or embarrassed. The indignity of illness has erased my sense of shame. I have willed that I can only feel bad about myself if I have been a hurtful jackass to another person.

Carl Jung said that "the word 'happiness' would lose its meaning if it were not balanced by sadness." We all have a finite amount of time, a limited amount of energy. It is up to us to make the most of it. The job of our lives is to work out who we are and work on becoming the best version of ourselves. It's never too late to get smarter or stronger.

Having strength does not mean you are not afraid. It means you have the guts to face what you fear. As Hemingway wrote, "The world breaks everyone and afterward many are strong at the broken places."

I have a serious illness, but I don't have to take it seriously. I have found an upside in having my life turned upside down. I have learned acceptance and resilience and have created a whole new life. In short, I grew a backbone.

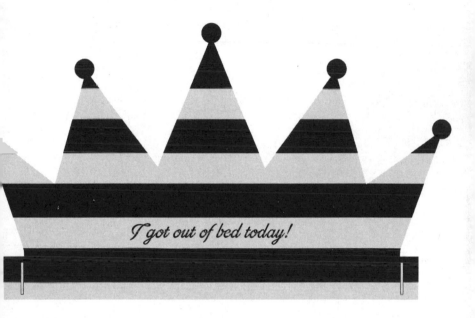

I got out of bed today!

GOT OUT OF BED TODAY CROWN

Instructions

Cut out slots, feed ribbon through slots and tie around your head. Congratulations!

APPENDIX:
THE HOLMES AND RAHE STRESS TEST

STRESS, LIKE PAIN, IS difficult to express with language. It's like pornography; as Supreme Court Justice Potter Stewart said, you know it when you see it. Each individual interprets stress differently, and it's difficult to communicate how we're suffering from stress, and how much.

The most widely accepted definition of stress, attributed to psychologist Richard S. Lazarus, is "a condition or feeling experienced when a person perceives that demands exceed the personal or social resources the individual is able to mobilize." More plainly, we feel stressed when we feel like things are out of our control.

The Holmes and Rahe Stress Test is self-assessment tool that helps us to identify the stresses in our life and understand the total burden of stress. The higher the score, the more likely you are to become ill, as stress is linked to health problems. For people with chronic conditions it's especially important to be aware of how stress might impact your already compromised health.

The scale is easy to use. Just go through the list, and give yourself points for every one of these events that has occurred in your life in the past year. Give yourself multiple points for multiple events—if you get locked up in the hoosegow twice, give yourself double points.

Rank	Life event	Mean value
1	Death of spouse	100
2	Divorce	73
3	Marital separation	65
4	Jail term	63
5	Death of close family member	63
6	Personal injury or illness	53
7	Marriage	50
8	Fired at work	47
9	Marital reconciliation	45
10	Retirement	45
11	Change in health of family member	44
12	Pregnancy	40
13	Sex difficulties	39
14	Gain of new family member	39
15	Business readjustment	39
16	Change in financial state	38
17	Death of close friend	37
18	Change to different line of work	36
19	Change in number of arguments with spouse	35
20	Mortgage over $10,000	31
21	Foreclosure of mortgage or loan	30
22	Change in responsibilities at work	29
23	Son or daughter leaving home	29
24	Trouble with in-laws	29
25	Outstanding personal achievement	28
26	Wife begin or stop work	26
27	Begin or end school	26
28	Change in living conditions	25
29	Revision of personal habits	24
30	Trouble with boss	23
31	Change in work hours or conditions	20
32	Change in residence	20
33	Change in schools	20
34	Change in recreation	19
35	Change in church activities	19
36	Change in social activities	18
37	Mortgage or loan less than $10,000	17
38	Change in sleeping habits	16
39	Change in number of family get-togethers	15
40	Change in eating habits	15
41	Vacation	13
42	Christmas	12
43	Minor violations of the law	11

Score of 300 or more: At risk of illness.
Score of 150-299: Moderate risk of illness
Score under 150: Slight risk of illness.

APPENDIX 2:
THE MCGILL PAIN SURVEY

THE TRADITIONAL VITAL SIGNS—INDICATORS of a person's health—are body temperature, blood pressure, heart rate, and breathing rate. As pain management and treatment has grown, a patent's type of pain is now regarded as a fifth vital sign.

The McGill Pain Questionnaire is a self-assessment test that helps you verbally express the sensation of pain. You select the words that best reflect your pain. When completed, you will have a short list of seven words that best express your pain. While originally published by Guilford Press in the *Handbook of Pain Assessment, Third Edition*, the McGill Pain Questionnaire can be found online in the *Journal of the American Society of Anethesiologists* at anesthesiology.pubs.asahq.org

ACKNOWLEDGMENTS

I'M DEEPLY APPRECIATIVE TO my esteemed colleagues for their editing, research, and encouragement. Francis Gasparini is the spine of this book. I am enormously grateful to work with him as his guidance, wisdom, and humor is evident on every page. Jim Duffy's rigorous copyediting made me appear smarter. Chelsea Domaleski's illustrations and contributions enhanced every chapter. David Kuhn and William LoTurco kept the faith at Aevitas Creative. Beth Canova, Caitlin Thomas, and Brian Peterson are a testament to the sterling professionalism at Arcade Publishing. Jeannette Seaver, my editor at Arcade Publishing, is my hero. The immensity of my gratitude for her faith in *Backbone* cannot be contained on a page.

One of my favorite quotes is from Ecclesiastics 6:16: "A faithful friend is the medicine of life." My thanks to Kate Firrioli, Laura Duffy, Lynn Fischer, Lori Campbell, Greg Shano, Peg Donegan, Lizzie Bracco, Andrew Muscato, Carole Radziwill, Megan Wilson, Kate Doege, Sara Story, Melissa Berger, Leigh Haber, the friend who chose the alias Francine Fishpaw, George Clooney, Bill Murray, Fr. Andrew Small, Amy

Sacco, Beautiful Jenny, Sara and Tim Geary, Joanna Molloy, Aida Turturro, Victoria Kennedy, Karim Chehimi, and Breena Whitcomb. You are my medicine, thanks.